Helga Bruxel Carvalho Follmann
Eliana E. Diehl

Indigenous people as nursing workers

Helga Bruxel Carvalho Follmann
Eliana E. Diehl

Indigenous people as nursing workers

Professionalization of the Kaingáng Indians in the west of Santa Catarina

ScienciaScripts

Imprint

Any brand names and product names mentioned in this book are subject to trademark, brand or patent protection and are trademarks or registered trademarks of their respective holders. The use of brand names, product names, common names, trade names, product descriptions etc. even without a particular marking in this work is in no way to be construed to mean that such names may be regarded as unrestricted in respect of trademark and brand protection legislation and could thus be used by anyone.

Cover image: www.ingimage.com

This book is a translation from the original published under ISBN 978-3-639-89887-3.

Publisher:
Sciencia Scripts
is a trademark of
Dodo Books Indian Ocean Ltd. and OmniScriptum S.R.L publishing group

120 High Road, East Finchley, London, N2 9ED, United Kingdom
Str. Armeneasca 28/1, office 1, Chisinau MD-2012, Republic of Moldova, Europe
Printed at: see last page
ISBN: 978-620-5-80855-9

I dedicate this work first of all to my husband Eric for being my partner, my companion, my friend who supports me in all my ventures and challenges that arise. This work and this stage were only possible due to his help and support.

My daughters Morgana and Sofia, who helped me to complete it, understanding my absences and supporting me.

To the Kaingáng people who received me with great affection.

Thank you

To my parents, Francisco and Sara for their help with the care of my daughters while I was living in the village, and simply for everything To my sister Silvia and my brother Rafael for their encouragement.

To my family members, brothers, brothers-in-law, uncles, father-in-law and mother-in-law who also helped in this journey, sometimes encouraging, sometimes supporting.

To my supervisor, Eliana Diehl, for her patience and guidance.

To the kaingáng for the warm reception, affection and help. To Matilde and her beloved family who welcomed me with open arms and saw me experience beautiful and unforgettable moments. To the chief who authorized my research, and who allowed my stay in the village.

To the nursing technicians and assistants who helped me a lot in this research by letting me accompany them in their work and to the health teams of the villages Sede, Pinhalzinho, Paiol de Barro and Fazenda São José who allowed me to accompany them in their work. The teachers for receiving me and answering my questions.

FUNASA and FUNAI who authorized my entry into the area to carry out this research.

To the professors of the Postgraduate Program in Collective Health. To CAPES for the scholarship. To the Brasil Plural National Research Institute for funding the field research.

I thank my guides, Mama Oxum and all the Orixás.

Thank you all!

"It is possible to disagree with the person and still love them. It is not necessary to make war with whom we do not agree. Kardec did it this way: he repudiated the opinion of his contradictors, but never disrespected the human being" *Spirit Zezinho*

"The difficulty in living together in society lies in man's conception that 'his' way of thinking is the right one ... In fact, there are no 'right' or 'wrong', only different points of view for each situation, and learning to respect and understand these 'other truths' can truly be the beginning of everything. We should not 'impose *our* right' on others, but try to adapt it, to the reality experienced, seeking the welfare of all."

Helga Follmann

SUMMARY

TITLE: Indigenous people as nursing workers: the role of technicians and assistants in the indigenous health care model

Indigenous health care has been undergoing changes over the last decades. From August 1999, the model was reconfigured into a Health Care Subsystem that is part of the Unified Health System, based on the National Policy for Health Care for Indigenous Peoples. This Subsystem incorporated the principle of differentiated attention, which advocates, among other things, the insertion of indigenous populations in the context of care through indigenous health agents (AIS), who have the role of being the link between the community and health teams and between local indigenous knowledge and biomedicine. As a reflection of the insertion of HIAs in the Multidisciplinary Team of Basic Indigenous Health Care, in some Indigenous Lands, the indigenous people are seeking greater professional qualification in health care. This research aimed to investigate the role of the indigenous nursing assistant/technician in the model of indigenous health care, identifying the profile, training and activities of these professionals. The research was carried out in the Xapecó Indigenous Land, Santa Catarina, in January and February 2011, using the ethnographic method, especially participant observation and semi-structured interviews. In the Xapecó Indigenous Land, there are currently 16 indigenous persons with secondary education in nursing, the majority Kaingáng, of whom ten work in a function compatible with their education. Of the 13 indigenous nursing technicians, ten started and completed a free course promoted by the Federal University of Santa Catarina (UFSC), called "Projeto Pioneiro" (Pioneer Project). The three indigenous nursing assistants completed free courses through the Professionalization of Nursing Workers Project (Profae) at the National Service for Commercial Learning (Senac) (two indigenous people) and the Professional Qualification Supplementary Course for Nursing Assistants, Braga, RS (one indigenous person). The activities performed by indigenous nursing assistants and technicians do not differ in practice: they are the same activities required of non-indigenous professionals of the same category. However, they also assume the function of facilitator, translator and interlocutor between the health team and the community. The team perceives them as the interlocutor of medical recommendations, curative, as well as the anxieties and fears of patients who do not want to undergo some medical procedure. The indigenous technician and auxiliary intervenes in order to make the patient and/or their carer accept and comply with the biomedical recommendation. The community, in turn, generally seeks the assistance of indigenous professionals, because "being Indians, they understand Indians". The data indicates the difficulty of articulation between the local knowledge of health and the biomedical model, since the indigenous technicians and assistants carry out their technical activities based on their biomedical training, leaving little or no space in the context of the health posts for other practices, such as the use of plants and home remedies. As the training courses maintain a biomedical curriculum base, with little time allocated to local knowledge and regional studies, it is a challenge to restructure the curricula and the health services in order to contemplate the Kaingáng knowledge and practices in health.

Key-words: indigenous health; nursing auxiliaries; South American Indians; Kaingáng Indians; health services.

ABSTRACT

The indigenous health care has undergone changes over the past decades. From August 1999, the model was reconfigured into a health care subsystem part of the National Health Care System, based on the National Policy for Health Care of Indigenous Peoples. This subsystem incorporates the principle of special care, which advocates, among others, the inclusion of indigenous peoples in the context of care through indigenous health agents (AIS), who have the role of being the link between community and health teams and among local indigenous knowledge and biomedicine. As a reflex to the inclusion of AIS in the Indigenous Health Primary Care Multidisciplinary Team, it is observed, in some Indigenous Lands, the search for a higher professional qualification in health by the indigenous. This research aimed to investigate the role of the indigenous nursing assistant/technician in the model of the indigenous health care, identifying the profile, formation and activities of these professionals. The research was held at the Xapecó Indigenous Land, in Santa Catarina, in January and February 2011, using the ethnographic method, especially the participant observation and the conduction of semi-structured interviews. On the Xapecó Indigenous Land there are currently 16 indigenous trained in nursing at high school level, most Kaingáng, and ten of them work in positions consistent to training. Among the 13 indigenous nursing technicians, ten started and completed a free course sponsored by the Federal University of Santa Catarina/UFSC, called "Pioneer Project". The three indigenous nursing assistants completed free courses by the Project of Professionalization of Workers in the Nursing Area/PROFAE at the National Service of Commercial Training /SENAC (two indigenous) and by the Nursing Assistant Professional Qualification Equivalency Course, in Braga, RS (one indigenous). The activities carried out by the indigenous nursing assistants and technicians do not differ in practice, being the same activities required of the non-indigenous professional from the same category. However, they still assume the role of facilitator, translator and interlocutor between the health team and community. The team perceives him as interlocutor of medical advice, healing, as well as the anxieties and fears of patients who do not want to perform some medical procedure. The indigenous technician and assistant intervene in order to make the patient and /or his/her caretaker agrees and meets the biomedical recommendation. The community, in turn, often seeks for indigenous professional assistance, because "being Indians, understand Indians". The data indicates the difficulty between local health knowledge and the biomedical model, since the indigenous technicians and assistants carry out their technical activities based on their biomedical training, leaving little or no space in the context of health clinics to other practices, such as the use of herbal plants and homemade remedies. As the training courses maintain a biomedical curricular basis, with little workload allocated to local knowledge and regional studies, it is a challenge to restructure curricula and health services in order to apply the Kaingáng knowledge and practices in health.

Keywords: Indigenous Health; Nursing Assistants; South American Indians; Kaingáng Indians; Health Services.

LIST OF ABBREVIATIONS

AIS - Indigenous Health Agent

AISAN - Indigenous Sanitation Agent

DSEI - Special Indigenous Health District

EMSI - Multidisciplinary Indigenous Health Team

EVS - Floating Health Teams

FUNAI - National Indian Foundation

FUNASA - National Health Foundation

IBGE - Brazilian Institute of Geography and Statistics

PNASPI - National Policy for Health Care for Indigenous Peoples

PROFAE - Professionalization Programme for Nursing Workers

RET-SUS - Network of Technical Schools of the Unified Health System

SENAC - National Commercial Learning Service

SIASI - Indigenous Health Care Information System SPI - Indian Protection Service

IT - Indigenous Land

SUMMARY

Introduction

The provision of health actions and services to indigenous peoples has undergone major modifications over the last few decades, with the landmark being in 1999, when the Ministry of Health granted the National Health Foundation (Funasa) responsibility for the Indigenous Health Care Subsystem, instituting the National Policy for Health Care for Indigenous Peoples (PNASPI) (BRASIL, 2002), recommended in the Brazilian Constitution of 1988 and in the Organic Health Law (Law no.° 8.080/1990). The Indigenous Health Care Subsystem is an integral part of the Unified Health System (SUS), aimed at differentiated care for indigenous peoples. It is executed through the Special Indigenous Health Districts (DSEI), and their implementation (34 DSEI in total) occurred at the end of 1999, promoting the hiring of health professionals to carry out primary care in the villages on Indigenous Lands and in the Base-Poles. The Polos-Base and, when possible, the village health posts house a Multidisciplinary Team for Basic Indigenous Health Care (EMSI), composed of the Basic Nucleus for Indigenous Health Care and the District Nucleus for Indigenous Health Care. The first is responsible for implementing the basic actions of indigenous health care and is made up of health professionals such as nurses, nursing auxiliaries or technicians, doctors, dentists, dental assistants, dental hygiene technicians, indigenous health agents, indigenous sanitation agents, sanitation technicians, endemic disease agents and microscopists in the Legal Amazon Region. The second is responsible for the execution of the actions of integral attention to the health of the indigenous population, composed of professionals who work in indigenous health, not contemplated in the composition referred to in the first Nucleus, such as nutritionists, pharmacists/biochemists, anthropologists, social workers and others, in view of the specific needs of the indigenous population (BRASIL, 2007).

Ideally, the EMSI should offer differentiated health care in the Indigenous Lands. The differentiated attention, officially understood as a differentiation in the quality of services, is given by the time of permanence in the indigenous area performing primary health care, i.e., prevention of diseases, basic care in clinical and emergency care. This differentiated attention is also proposed as an articulation between indigenous health knowledge and practices and the biomedical model, thus respecting the social, cultural, political and economic dimensions of each ethnic group (LANGDON and DIEHL, 2007).

However, recent work shows that EMSI members are generally unprepared to deal with the different cultures with which they interact in the work process in indigenous communities. Langdon et al. (2006); Langdon and Diehl (2007); Mendonça (2005); Garnelo et al. (2003), among others, show that differentiated care is far from becoming a reality and point out that one of the main difficulties lies in the lack of education and training of health professionals to act in specific interethnic contexts.

In the context of indigenous health, a gradual increase of indigenous people seeking training and working as nursing technicians or assistants is observed. Research in Santa Catarina (LANGDON et al., 2006; LANGDON and DIEHL, 2007) also evidences that many were taking courses as nursing auxiliaries or technicians, or even concluding high school, as a way to ascend professionally, since the Subsystem created an important demand for jobs in the Indigenous Lands. However, there are still no studies that focus on these workers, contrary to what has been observed in relation to research on Indigenous Health Agents (see, for example, MENDONÇA, 2005; LANGDON et al., 2006; DIAS-SCOPEL, 2008; MARINHO and OTT, 2007; NOVO, 2008), which highlight that the definitions about the role of the AIS and the evaluations of their work reveal ambiguities and tensions that emerge from their relations with their own indigenous peers and with their non-indigenous peers.

At EMSI, the nursing technician/assistant, after the AIS, is the professional who has the greatest contact with the population. This professional has more complex activities than the agent, such as the intravenous, intramuscular and intradermal application of medicines, distribution of medicines, application of vaccines, dressings, etc. In some cases, the technician/indigenous assistant assumes the local coordination of health posts, as among the Xokleng of Santa Catarina.

According to Ribeiro and Pedrão (2005), the care model performed by technicians and nursing auxiliaries is technicist and uncritical reproduction of existing practices. In this sense, investigating how the indigenous technicians and auxiliaries have appropriated the biomedical knowledge and acted facing the health demands of the population is relevant, as it may provide subsidies to effect differentiated care. It should be noted that the National Policy for the Health Care of Indigenous Peoples (BRASIL, 2002) particularly highlights the HIA as the fundamental link for the articulation between indigenous knowledge and biomedical knowledge, without emphasizing other indigenous professionals who can also be key players in this articulation.

Despite the fact that the Subsystem has been in operation for some years, studies on the adequacy of training and capacity building courses for acting in intercultural situations are rare. Such research is essential to support public policies, the training of human resources to act in intercultural contexts and, consequently, the improvement of the quality of services.

In this sense, this study aimed to analyze the role, in the model of indigenous health care, of the indigenous worker trained as a nursing assistant or technician, identifying their profile, the courses taken, the activities developed, as well as their perception, that of the community and the team on the insertion in the EMSI of the Xapecó Indigenous Land, Santa Catarina.

This work culminating in this research spans the journey I have travelled.

I worked with all the aspects that involved this research. Initially, as a nurse, I worked as a nurse in the Family Health Programme, then as a teacher and coordinator of nursing technical courses, I also worked in the state secretariat of Paraná as a supervisor of nursing technical courses and in indigenous health as a nurse and coordinator, thus having a broad view of the whole context. However, the need for answers made me seek a Master's degree in Public Health in order to try to answer some questions. Initially, a literature review is made, pointing out aspects considered important for the understanding and discussion of the theme, including history, geographical location and sociocultural information about the Kaingáng, based on works already written about this group, and the current organization of the health care model. After that, the trajectory of the researcher in indigenous health and the process of conducting the research, which is characterized as a qualitative, descriptive study, is briefly described. The results of the research itself are presented in the chapter "The insertion of indigenous people as nursing workers," in which the indigenous people with training as nursing assistants or technicians are identified, describing and analyzing their profile, training and activities, seeking to understand their role in the EMSI and in the organization of health care in the Xapecó Indigenous Land, in dialogue with the aspects previously reviewed. In the final considerations, we seek to resume the main results of the research and reflect on its contribution to indigenous health.

CHAPTER 1

1. Reviewing the literature

1.1 The Kaingáng

1.1.1 Background

The process of colonisation of Brazil is marked by many struggles, conflicts and bloodshed. The indigenous peoples who lived here before the arrival of the Portuguese colonizers lived in conflicts between the various existing ethnic groups or even between groups of the same ethnic group. After the contact of Indians with non-Indians, the conflicts continued, often stimulated by the non-Indians with the intention of subjugating some ethnic group or groups of Indians in a certain region, sometimes with the intention of reducing the strength of the local ethnic group, in order to gain possession of the land (TOMMASINO, 2000).

It is estimated that when the colonisers arrived here the indigenous population was approximately three million people. The Brazilian Institute of Geography and Statistics (IBGE) estimated by the 2000 Census (the 2010 Census data for indigenous populations is not yet available) that this population was reduced to a little over 400,000 Indians still living in villages throughout Brazil (BRASIL, 2000). The so-called "aldeados" Indians, that is, those who still live in the villages, receive differentiated health actions and services, as discussed below.

Brazil has approximately 215 different ethnic groups, speaking 180 languages distributed in 30 linguistic families. It is believed that there are about 55 groups of isolated Indians, of which there is still no information (BRASIL, 2005, p. 15).

According to FUNAI[1] , the view of indigenous people is sometimes prejudiced and sometimes idealised. The idea that the indigenous people occupy the land without using it, that it would be a "waste to leave so much land to those who produce nothing" and that the indigenous people hinder the progress of the country is unfortunately part of an old but not outdated vision, which is still present today. It is in rural areas that strong prejudice is perceived due to direct contact with indigenous people and the struggle for land and environmental resources. Often, stereotypes such as "thieves", "lazy", "treacherous" and "drunkards" are used to disqualify them and thus try to justify all kinds of actions against indigenous peoples and the invasion of their territories. On the other hand, the population living in the cities tends to have a "romanticized" view of the Indians, idealizing them as the first inhabitants of the nation, beings who live in communion with nature and do not depredate it.

1.1.2 Who are the Kaingáng?

The Kaingáng represent one of the five most numerous indigenous populations in Brazil, with 33,876 individuals (BRASIL, 2010) who are distributed across São Paulo, Paraná, Rio Grande do Sul and 6,397 in Santa Catarina.

Reports by Nimuendajú (1993 [1919]) and Telêmaco Borba (1902 [1882]) describe the linguistic issue of the Kaingáng. At the time, they were also called crowned, and were often confused with the Xokleng. Their language, studied for more than 100 years, belongs to the Macro-Jê linguistic trunk, the most spoken in Brazil (for more details, see D'Angelis, 1989 and Noelli, 1998, who deal with the Macro-Jê languages).

Nimuendajú (1993 [1919]), in his conviviality with the Kaingáng (1910-1912), observed the confrontation of opinions about indigenous populations. On the one hand, the extermination of the "savages" who would impede progress and civilization; and on the other, positions such as that of the humanist Rondon, who fought for the respect of these peoples and their cultures.

The history of resistance of the Kaingáng to domination by non-Indians, the armed conflicts in the struggle for possession of their land, the intervention of the Indian Protection Service (SPI) and the removal from the Kaingáng lands are well described in the works by D'Angelis (1989), Mota et al. (2000) and Nacke et al. (2007) on a history marked by many conflicts and interactions with the surrounding society. This becomes visible when observing the Indigenous Land (T.I. Xapecó), which in 1902 had approximately 50,000 hectares when the SPI was created in 1910, and today has approximately 15,000 hectares (SANTOS, 1979). The SPI played an important role in this territorial decrease, as employees of this organ intervened as mediators between ranchers and indigenous people, not always helping the indigenous people. This decrease occurred due to land appropriation by immigrants, who, in "agreement" with the indigenous people, planted the crops and offered them jobs in the plantations. However, after some time, the lands were claimed by the European immigrants (NACKE et al., 2007). With the frequent contact between Indians and non-Indians, the Portuguese language was being learned. Today, in the Indigenous Lands inhabited by the Kaingáng, Portuguese is widely spoken, which in some cases is the predominant language.

The old people can still converse in their native language, and children are being re-educated in their native language, mainly through bilingual literacy. The retaking of the language is an important element for the legitimization of their culture. However, being Kaingáng is much more than just speaking the language. After so many years of contact, it is common to hear from populations living close to the indigenous populations that there are no more Indians, but "caboclos" who want to pass themselves off as Indians to receive government benefits, in an attempt to demean the local indigenous people. For the Kaingáng, to **be** Kaingáng is related to the land, place where they live, family/ ancestors, customs and, recently, with the resumption of the mother tongue to legitimize their identity:

> The situation in relation to the language spoken varies from one land to another: there are communities where all are Kaingáng speakers, in others they are Portuguese speakers with the exception of the elders who are bilingual and in others, the majority of the population are bilingual or Portuguese speakers. Even with these variations one notices that the Kaingáng, in general, have come to value the use of the mother tongue as an important element, politically, to affirm the legitimacy of their struggles for land (TOMMASINO and FERNANDES, 2001)[2]

1.1.3 Some ethnographic data

Kaingáng, Caingangue or Kaingangue were formerly called crowned because of their haircut. Etymologically, their name means people from the bush (TOMMASINO, 2000). This name was given to them by Telêmaco Borba, in 1882, to differentiate them from the Guarani and Xokleng who lived nearby (SIMIEMA, 2000)[3].

The Kaingáng vision of world creation begins with two Kaingáng who took refuge inside the earth when there was the great flood throughout the world. After the flood ceased, the two Kaingáng came out from inside the earth. One came out on the dry side of the hole and the other on the wet side. The one that came out on the dry side represents the *Kamé:* the sun, the hot, the strong, the bright, symbolized by "streaks/lines"; the one that came out on the wet side of the earth, the mud, is the *Kairu:* the moon, the cold, the humid, the weak, symbolized by the "round/circle" (OLIVEIRA, 1996; ALMEIDA, 2004).

Thus, the world would be divided between the *Kamé* and the *Kairu:* plants, animals, food and the Kaingáng themselves. They are two halves that complete each other, and marriages usually take place between the exogamous halves[4] . This means that the marriage occurs between two complementary opposite halves and, after the marriage, the daughters live close to their family, that is, the women of the family group, mothers and daughters, are always close to each other, and the husband has to accompany his wife to the proximities of her family. The descent is patrilineal, that is, the children inherit half of what belongs to the father. There are several works that describe in more detail the Kaingáng cosmological division into *Kamé* and *Kairu,* such as Baldus (1937), among others more recent, such as Fernandes (1998) and Almeida (2004). Other, more current works also bring descriptions about the Kaingáng on various topics: health, healing rituals and shamanism (GARCIA, 2010; ROCHA, 2005; ROSA, 2005;

DIEHL, 2001a; DIEHL, 2001b; FASSHEBER, 2003; OLIVEIRA, 1996), ethnobotany (HAVERROTH, 1997), territory and territoriality (MOTA et al, 2000), Kaingáng politics (FERNANDES, 1998), church and religion (ALMEIDA, 2004), food and culture (OLIVEIRA, 2009), among others.

The *Kiki* ritual[5] , also called the ritual of the dead, is the most expressive rite of this ethnic group. In this ritual, the dead are divided between *Kamé* and *Kairú,* and it is necessary that the dead include people from both halves. This ritual is a great celebration between the living and the dead, in which the social organisation and the Kaingáng world view can be perceived.

1.1.4 Geographic location of the Kaingáng

The Kaingáng are one of the most numerous indigenous peoples in Brazil, located in Indigenous Lands in São Paulo, Paraná, Santa Catarina and Rio Grande do Sul. However, despite the land demarcations, the Kaingáng move between their lands, from São Paulo to Rio Grande do Sul, without being disturbed by demarcation issues made by non-Indians, as they believe that the land belongs to them and that they are free to move between them.

> Kaingáng territory is also the space where the spirits of their ancestors and other supernatural beings dwell. It is where their dead are buried and where the living have their navels buried. In the rituals of the dead (kiki koi), the spirits of the dead return to commune with the living. The indigenous concept of territory thus gains a socio-political and cosmological dimension that is much broader than that of whites. (...) the Kaingáng produced their territories according to their own concept of time and space. The Kaingáng way of life implies a specific relationship with nature and with each other, according to historically developed symbolic representations that give meaning to their material and social practices. Being and becoming human is related to living according to the practical and symbolic Kaingáng model (TOMMASINO, 2000, pp. 210-211).

Transition between the villages and indigenous lands is quite common, whether to visit relatives, look for partners, work and/or sell handicrafts, as well as to change for political and/or economic reasons.

In Santa Catarina (Figure 1), the Kaingáng are found in the T.I. Xapecó, Chimbangue I and II, Pinhal, Condá, Toldo Imbu (in process of demarcation) and also on the border with Paraná (T.I. Palmas) (NACKE et al., 2007).

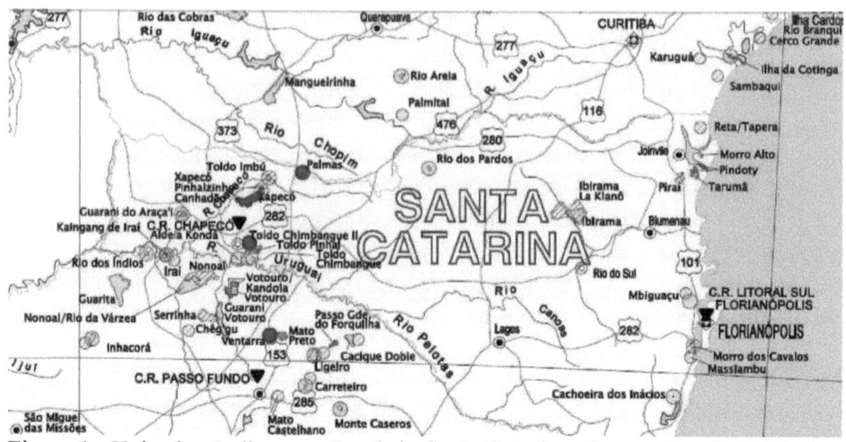

Figure 1 - Kaingáng Indigenous Lands in Santa Catarina. Source: Brazil (2011 a).

1.1.5 Xapecó Indigenous Land[6]

The demarcation of the T.I. Xapecó began in 1934 by the State Government of Santa Catarina and the SPI after heated conflicts over land ownership between Kaingángs and non-Indians. Through the Decree n° 46, of 11 July 1934, the State Government determined that the indigenous lands and their demarcations were respected in the municipality of Chapecó for the use of Indians. In 1952, through an agreement with the SPI and the Directorate of Land and Colonization of the State, new boundaries were defined for the region, which initially was 25 thousand hectares. The measurement and demarcation of the land in 1987 defined 15,623 hectares for the T.I. Xapecó, which was ratified by Decree No.º 297 of 29 October 1991[7] (NOTZOLD, 2004, p. 5).

Currently, the T.I. Xapecó is located "in the municipalities of Ipuaçu and Entre Rios (Figure 2), located in the western mesoregion of Santa Catarina, and corresponds to approximately 40% of the total extension of these municipalities" (NACKE et al., 2007, p. 43).

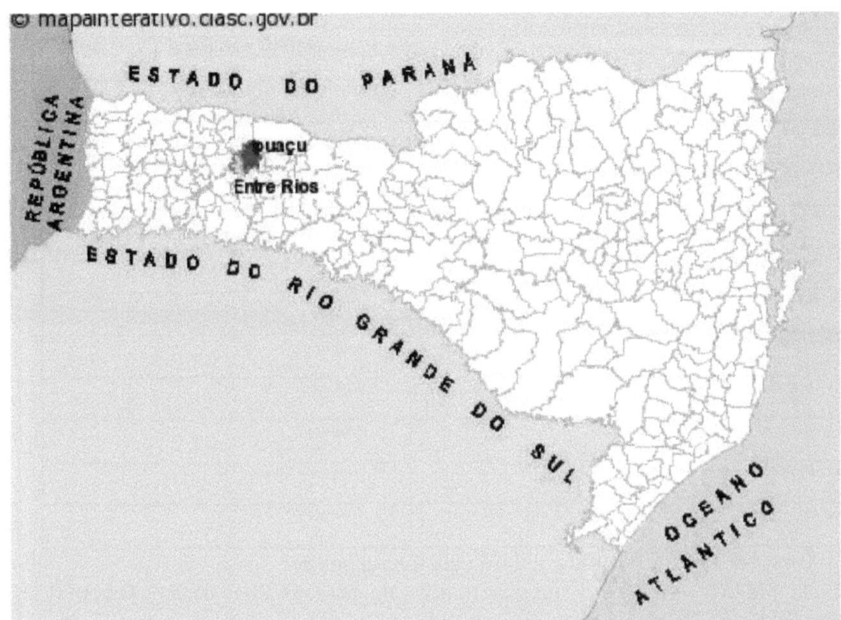

Figure 2 - Location of the Xapecó Indigenous Land, in the cities of Ipuaçu and Entre Rios, Santa Catarina. Adapted from: <http://www.mapainterativo. ciasc.gov.br/sc.phtml>. Accessed on: 12 May 2011.

The villages belonging to the T.I. Xapecó (Figure 3) are described in Table 1, and of the 212 inhabitants of the village Limeira, 102 are Guarani Indians.

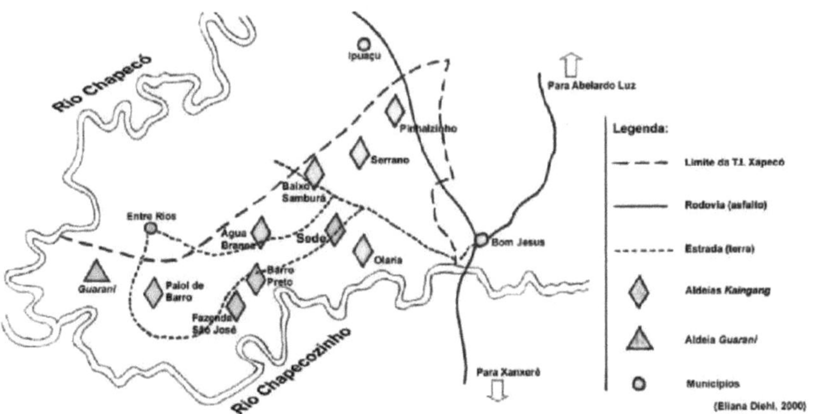

Figure 3 - Croquis of the T. I. Xapecó, Santa Catarina. Source: Diehl (2001b, p. 35).

Table 1: Villages of the Xapecó Indigenous Land and respective populations.

Village	Population (n)°	Located in the municipality
Headquarters	1.538	Ipuaçu
Pinhalzinho	1.183	Ipuaçu
White Water	285	Ipuaçu
São José Farm	102	Ipuaçu
Serrano	58	Ipuaçu
Serro Doce	104	Ipuaçu
Pottery	295	Ipuaçu
Bass Samburá	299	Ipuaçu
Serrano	68	Ipuaçu
Clay magazine	578	Between Rivers
Limeira	212	Between Rivers

Source: Brazil (2010). Available at: <http://sis.funasa.gov.br/ transparencia_publica/siasiweb/Layout/quantitativo_de_pessoas_2010.asp#>. Accessed on: 15 mar. 2011.

Figures 4, 5 and 6 show some aerial images that illustrate the Xapecó IT.

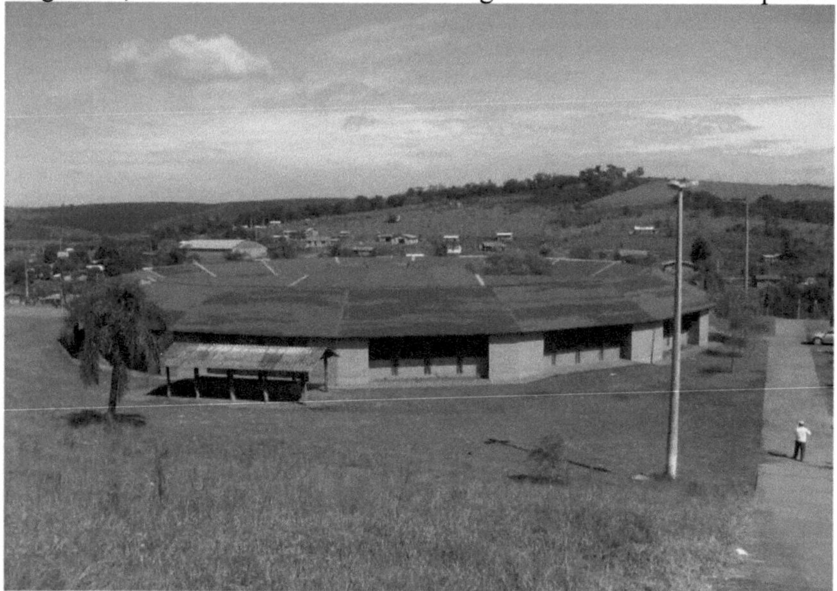

Figure 4 - Image of part of the village Headquarters: classrooms of the Cacique Vanhkre Indigenous School of Basic Education, T.I. Xapecó (Photo courtesy of an indigenous nursing technician).

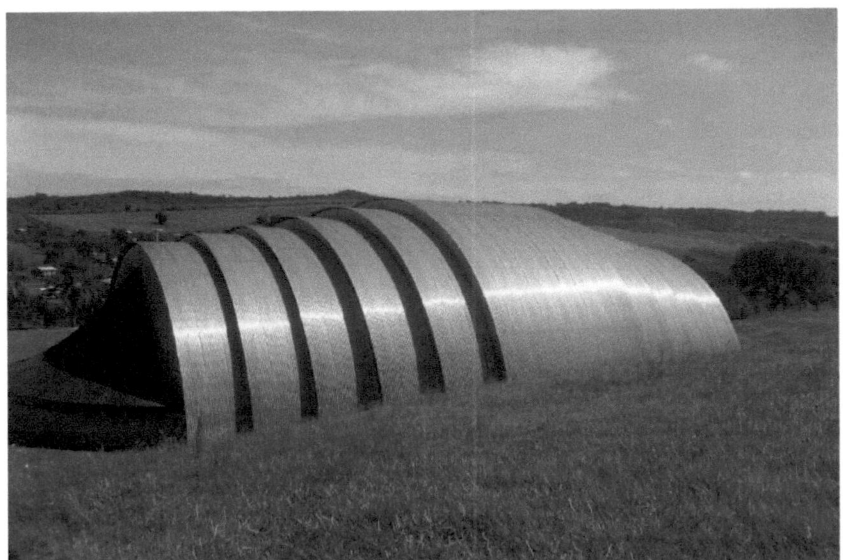

Figure 5 - Image of part of the village Headquarters: Sports gymnasium in armadillo shape/Indigenous School of Basic Education Cacique Vanhkre, T.I. Xapecó.

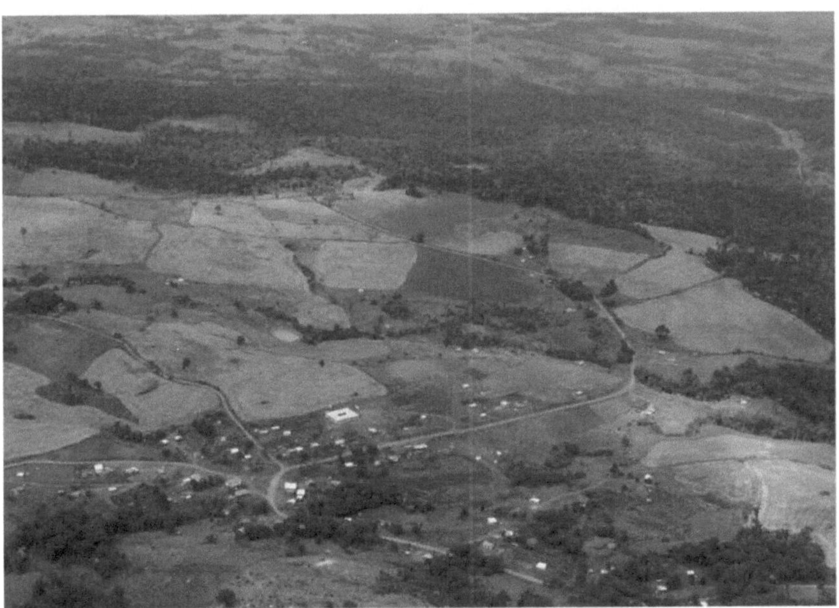

Figure 6 - Aerial view of the Paiol de Barro village, Xapecó IT.

In the past, subsistence was provided by hunting, gathering (mainly of fruits, such as pine nuts) and fishing, which are still practiced today whenever possible (CASTRO, 2010). Currently the indigenous people work in the villages or outside them. In the T.I. Xapecó, for example, there is a pottery in the village of the same name, where some indigenous people work. There are also jobs generated by the health services, such as indigenous health and sanitation agents, nursing auxiliaries and technicians, general services assistants, drivers, and work in schools as teachers, school lunch ladies, etc. In the villages there are also jobs in the harvesting of beans, soya and maize (the latter two planted on a large scale by the local cooperative), as well as in small family businesses. The jobs outside the village are usually in the plantations, slaughterhouses and poultry farms near the T.I. Xapecó (TOMMASINO, 2000; DIEHL, 2001a).

It is common to plant corn, beans and pumpkin, among others, for subsistence.

> At first, the creation of the indigenous reserves allowed, in part, the continuity of the traditional Kaingáng model of subsistence. Very quickly, however, their traditional way of life was rendered unviable by the significant reduction in land and natural resources to which they had access, both in the areas officially reserved to them and in the spaces they managed to secure in the interstices of the lands acquired by the settlers. The destruction of the rivers made fish scarce. The Kaingáng continued to cultivate maize and other products in the traditional manner (NACKE et al., 2007, p. 39).

Their political organisation is centred on the Cacique, who is elected together with the vice-cacique by the community. It is up to them to resolve conflicts, organise undertakings, seek solutions to collective problems, such as issues related to health care. Together with the Indigenous Council, composed of former caciques and older people, meetings are held to deliberate on the actions to be taken, which may be of individual demands, as well as to resolve matters of general interest to the community (NACKE et al., 2007).

Moving house is quite common among the Kaingáng. Often the reason for dismantling the residence and rebuilding it just a few metres away may be due to a death in the family. However, nowadays many houses are made of bricks and cement and no longer of wood, making this practice more difficult.

Sanitation is still precarious, especially in the more remote villages: potable water and sewage are lacking in most houses. Even in the main village, the most structured, many houses do not have piped water and sewage. The T.I. Xapecó has an indigenous sanitation agent (AISAN) whose function is to provide families with guidance in the treatment of water, with the distribution of hypochlorite, and in hygiene, among other activities. Electricity supply is restricted to those who live in or near the large villages.

In the Xapecó Indigenous Territory there are schools in the villages of Sede (Escola Indígena de Educação Básica Cacique Vanhkre), Fazenda São José,

Pinhalzinho and Paiol de Barro. The school in the village Sede is the biggest of all and currently also offers secondary education in the evening timetable. There is a transport system between the villages to take and fetch the students to and from the schools.

Some residents have their own cars and motorbikes, usually bought used, which they use to go to the city, to college or to work, as well as for shopping and sightseeing. Even so, the vast majority need the bus as a means of transport. The buses from the meatpacking companies, which take the workers, are the most common, but there are also bus lines that can be used to the bus station of Xanxerê (about 30 km away from T.I.).

On religious questions, the Kaingáng are predominantly divided into Catholics and Evangelicals. The doctoral thesis of Ledson Kurtz de Almeida (2004) discusses the relationship of the various churches among the Kaingáng, showing that, despite the growth of the evangelical churches, the Catholic religion still plays an important role. The number of churches is large, and even where there are few houses, there are Evangelical Pentecostal churches.

1.2 Contextualising Indigenous Health

When it comes to indigenous health, it is known that many populations have been reduced or exterminated by diseases, especially infectious and contagious diseases. The Brazilian government was slow to assume responsibility for the care of these populations. The first steps occurred through the Indian Protection Service (SPI), starting in 1910 (BRASIL, 2011b), giving priority to Indians who came into contact with non-Indians. Later, FUNAI, which replaced the SPI in 1967, took over indigenous health, systematising the service to indigenous populations. There was a predominance of a welfare service through nursing attendants (often non-indigenous) in the interior of the indigenous areas and with the provision of medicines in the villages. The Equipes Volantes de Saúde (EVS - Mobile Health Teams) were also created, composed of a doctor, nurse, laboratorians and dentists, who periodically went to the villages to provide assistance in emergency cases. In the 1980s, the frequency of the EVS decreased until they were completely deactivated (NACKE et al., 2007, pp. 123-124).

After the 1st National Conference on the Protection of Indigenous Health in 1986, when indigenous health was specifically discussed, emphasis began to be placed on the creation of a differentiated model for indigenous peoples that respected their social, political and cultural dimensions, with the repercussions of this debate in the 1988 Constitution. Between 1991 and 1994, indigenous health care passed from FUNAI to the National Health Foundation (at the time FNS) (BRASIL, 1987), which created the Special Indigenous Health Districts (DSEI) as a Subsystem of the SUS, with only the DSEI Yanomami being created

(DIEHL, 2001a). Between 1994 and mid-1999, for political reasons, indigenous health was once again the responsibility of FUNAI. In August 1999, the Brazilian government took the decision to definitively transfer the actions and services of health to the Ministry of Health, more specifically to FUNASA. Thirty-four DSEI were then implanted throughout Brazil (Figure 7), which generated an increase in the hiring of health professionals to provide primary care in the villages on Indigenous Lands and in the Base Poles.

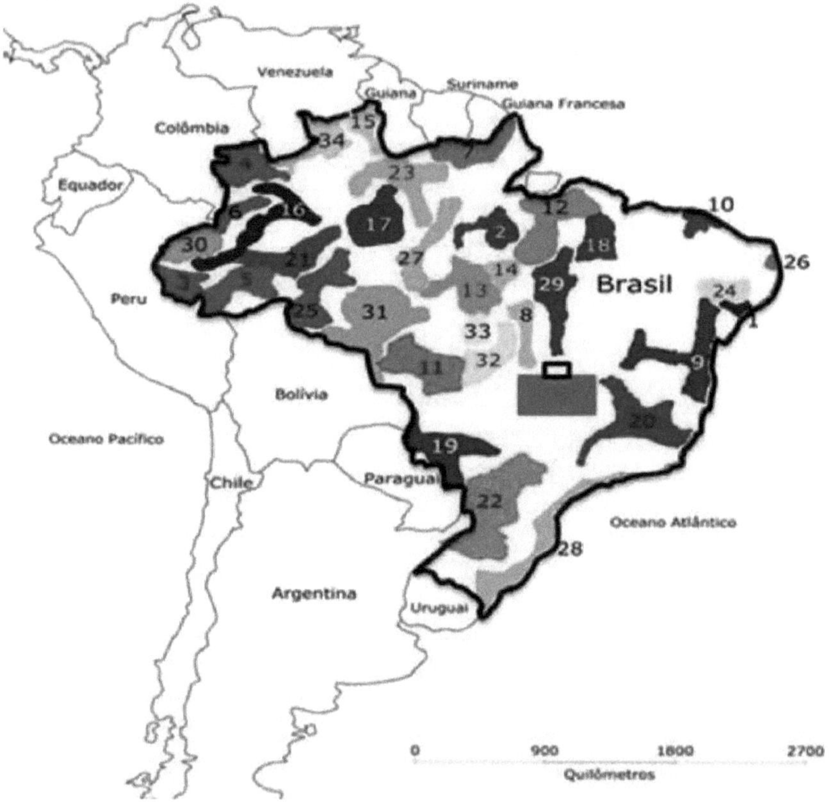

Figure 7 - Special Indigenous Health Districts. DSEI 22 corresponds to DSEI Interior Sul. Available at:
<http://portal.saude.gov.br/portal/ health/manager/area.cfm?id_area=1744>.

The DSEI must have instances of social control, which implies that health planning must be participatory and consider the population's own concepts of health and illness. This social control is the responsibility of the Local Health Councils, whose representatives are exclusively indigenous, and the District Health Councils, whose representation is made up of 50% indigenous people and 50% service providers, such as Non-Governmental Organisations (NGOs), town halls and health workers (DIEHL, 2001a).

Like the SUS, the Health Care Subsystem for Indigenous Peoples, articulated with the SUS, is decentralized, hierarchical, and universal, also including the principle of differentiated care. Primary or basic care takes place at the village level, where the actions of
disease prevention and health promotion are carried out by the EMSI, which also supervises the Indigenous Health Agent (AIS). The secondary and/or tertiary care services are activated in case there is an aggravation that requires specialized care or hospital intervention, that is, the patient will be taken to clinics and/or reference hospitals for consultation, treatment or hospitalization.

> The D SEI structure foresees that the majority of grievances are resolved in these two instances [villages or Polo-Base]. The demands that are not resolved at this level should be referred to specialized services at the headquarters of nearby municipalities or, depending on the case, to hospitals of low to high complexity and resolutivity. Furthermore, the Indian Houses, structures created by Funai, will be readapted to function as Indian Health Houses, serving as support between the villages and the SUS assistance network (DIEHL, 2001a, p. 43).

Despite the fact that the Subsystem has been active for approximately 11 years, little progress can be noted with regard to differentiated care. There is no consensus on how to implement or even evaluate it. According to Langdon et al. (2006, p. 29), "the National Policy on Health Care for Indigenous Peoples highlights the training of indigenous health agents as a central point to promote differentiated care, conceiving them as a link between traditional and biomedical knowledge", but studies have shown that the training and capacity building of these professionals, as well as the rest of the EMSI, is still very flawed (GARNELO et al., 2003; LANGDON et al., 2006; LANGDON and DIEHL, 2007).
According to the Situational Diagnosis of the Indigenous Health Subsystem (IDS/SSL/CEBRAP, 2009, p. 16):

> It is observed that there are national policies based on the principles of universality, integrality and equity that seek to reduce the differences in health conditions. However, there is little clarity about what a model of differentiated attention to indigenous health would be, prevailing the conception of the districts as an organisational model and practices centred on medical-curative procedures.

The allocation of financial resources for the subsystem is supplementary, made through fund-to-fund transfers from the central level to the municipalities whose municipalities have indigenous people in their territories and through agreements between FUNASA (which is gradually being replaced by the Special Secretariat for Indigenous Health) and universities (e.g., the Federal University of São Paulo) or indigenous or non-indigenous NGOs. The EMSI members can be hired directly by the municipalities or by those with agreements, generating different bonds that often have a negative impact on the work process of the team.

The Information System for Indigenous Health Care (SIASI) was created especially for the Subsystem, functioning through the accounting of the activities carried out by the EMSI in the villages and Base-Poles, which ideally should generate data that can serve as subsidies for the construction of indigenous health indicators and for the evaluation of the quality of life of the indigenous people and the health services (DIEHL, 2001a, p. 43). The SIASI "aims at the collection, processing and analysis of information for monitoring the health of indigenous communities, covering deaths, births, morbidity, immunization, production of services, human resources and infrastructure" (SOUSA et al., 2007, p. 854). However, as Sousa et al. (2007) point out, "the main limitations of the SIASI refer to the collection instruments, the training of human resources, the absence of an interface with the other national health information systems, the difficulty of access to the information and the non-use of the information for action planning" (p. 860).

On 19 October 2010, by means of Decree No.º 7.336, the Ministry of Health and FUNASA should effect the transition of the management of the Indigenous Health Care Subsystem to the Special Secretariat of Indigenous Health of the Ministry of Health, but the deadline was revoked until 31 December 2011 by Decree No.º 7.461 /2011 (BRASIL, 2011a).

The Indigenous Health Care Subsystem and the National Policy for Indigenous Peoples' Health Care place great emphasis on the role of indigenous health agents as members of the EMSI, who act as a link between the community and the team and between indigenous and biomedical knowledge. Such insertion is
based on documents and recommendations existing since the end of the 1970s, as will be seen below.

1.2.1 The insertion of members of the assisted communities in primary health care: Community Health Agents (CHAs) and Indigenous Health Agents (IHAs)

The World Health Organization (WHO), in the Alma-Ata Declaration (1978), recommends that primary health care should include, where applicable, at the local level, community agents, as well as traditional practitioners, as necessary, **properly trained socially and technically to work as a health team** (emphasis added) and respond to the expressed health needs of the community (WHO, 1978).[8]

Thus, among the urgent actions to protect and promote the health of all the people in the world, primary health care actions and services are needed, with community health workers residing in the communities where they will provide assistance, duly trained and technically able to develop health actions together with the team.

1.2.1.1 Community Health Agents

The Community Health Agent (CHA) appeared with the nomenclature of Sanitary Visitor and Sanitation Inspector at the beginning of the 20th century, a time of many endemics and epidemics, such as yellow fever. The first CHWs were called "barefoot doctors" in China in 1949 .[9]

Community health workers are part of the basic composition of the health team. As they are residents of the community where the team will operate, they are familiar with that community and its housing and sanitation conditions.

> It is believed that because they (the agents) are people's people, they not only resemble the characteristics and longings of these people, but also fill gaps, precisely because they know the needs of this population. I believe that agents are the springboard for the consolidation of the Unified Health System, the organisation of communities and the regionalised and hierarchical practice of care, in the structuring of health districts. Being a health agent is being a people, it's being a community, it's living day to day the life of that community (...) It's being the link between the population's health needs and what can be done to improve their living conditions. It's being the bridge between the population and health professionals and services. The community agent is the health messenger of his/her community (Head of the National Health Foundation, Brazil, 1991 apud SILVA e DALMASO, 2002, p. 5).

In Brazil, the ACS were part of the process of creating the Unified Health System, established by the Constitution in 1988, and were initially enrolled, in 1991, in the National Programme of Community Agents (PNAC). In 1992, the PNAC was renamed the Community Health Agents Programme (PACS), and the ACS were incorporated into the teams of the Family Health Programme (PSF) in 1994 (LANGDON et al., 2006).

The ACS occupation was created with the purpose of forming the link between the community and health professionals. This professional has to belong to the community where he/she will be working, as he/she is responsible for bringing information about the health conditions of the members, so that the health team is able to dimension the problems and plan their care actions. The recognition and incorporation of this professional occurred in 2002 through the Law nº 10.507 (BRASIL, 2002b). Their functions and activities are described in Law nº 11.350/2006, which regulates their hiring and their profession.

> Among the duties of CHWs defined by the Ministry of Health (MH), two deserve special attention when discussing the training of these professionals. The first states that CHWs must "guide families to the appropriate use of health services" and the second stresses that they must "inform other members of the health team about the social dynamics of the community, its availability and needs" (MH, 1998:18). Curiously, in these two attributions one can identify the bi-directional movement of the agents, those who, on the one hand, inform the population of "ways of doing" established by the official medical system and, on the other hand, provide health professionals with key elements for understanding the health problems of families and the needs of the population (NUNES et al., 2002, p. 1640).

They still lacked a training that would support their work, a certification. However, this action was complicated by the profile of CHWs, for whom setting up a technical course proved to be a challenge, as stated by Morosini and Corbo (2007):

> However, the operationalization of the technical level training of CHWs is not a simple task. This operationalization is faced with the complexities inherent to the very configuration of the CHWs' activity, with respect to the innovative nature of the activity, the fragility of their professional identity and incipient regulation. Furthermore, the training of CHWs transcends the health sector. Admittedly, the work of community health workers deals with issues related to citizenship, politics, living conditions and the organization of groups and their relationships, including the family (p. 12).

For Silva and Dalmaso (2002, p. 77), "historically, the idea that supports the insertion of the community health agent involves a concept that, under the most different forms, nomenclatures and rationalities, appear in various parts of the world, that is, the essential idea of link between the community and the health system" (p. 77). These authors further point out that:

> (...) as a community health agent, although with varying degrees of emphasis placed, it manages to

> It is possible to identify two main components or dimensions of its proposed action: one more strictly technical, related to

the care of individuals and families, the intervention for
prevention of diseases or for the monitoring of groups or
specific problems, and another more political, but not only of
solidarity with the population, of the insertion of health in the
general context of life, but also in the sense of community
organization, of transformation of these conditions (SILVA
and DALMASO 2002, p. 77).

Silva and Dalmaso (2002) observed that the agent suffers with his condition of meeting the community's expectations about health, as well as meeting the technical issues of the health team. The contradictions between meeting the community and the system to which he belongs are "the agent's permanent dilemma: the social dimension coexisting with the technical care dimension. By incorporating these two facets in their formulations, the conflict appears mainly in the dynamics of daily practice" (SILVA and DALMASO, 2002, p. 77).

In another study conducted by Silva (2001) (apud SILVA e DALMASO, 2002) on the community agent of the QUALIS/PSF Project, in the municipality of São Paulo, the author:

(...) identified that the community agent does not have the
tools, the technology, here included the knowledge for the
different dimensions expected of his work. This insufficiency
means that they end up working with common sense, with
religion and, more rarely, with the knowledge and resources
of families and the community. There is knowledge on loan
for the technical pole, but not for the dimension considered as
more political, nor are there proposals or consistent work of
'communicative action' (SILVA, 2001 apud SILVA e
DALMASO, 2002, p. 78).

This reflection is not intended to belittle the very important role of this professional, but to observe that not always the health team perceives him/her as a "knowledge carrier of the community". The activities of this professional of "monitoring" the actions of individuals to inform professionals about the "failure to follow medical guidelines" makes them "well seen" by the team, but not always by the community. On the other hand, professionals who stimulate the self-care of the community, instructing as to procedures and/or search for healers other than those of biomedicine[10] are also not "well accepted" by the health teams, who see in this professional someone who interferes and can "harm health actions".

In a recent study, Mota and David (2010) show the increasing schooling of CHWs added to collective mobilization and institutional motivation, derived from training policy, a process of certification by competence based on minimum education, referenced by the *Curricular Reference for Technical Course of Community Health Workers of the* Ministry of Health in 2004. This course is offered in the 36 networks of technical schools of the Unified Health System (RET-SUS) and is divided into three stages: I) initial training, which gives access to all CHWs who work in the SUS, regardless of schooling; II) completion of stage I who present the certificate of completion or certification of being in primary schools; III) completion of stage I and II who present the certificate of completion of high school or certification of completion concomitant with high school.

The authors point out that, although the Ministry of Health considers relevant the training of this professional who works closer to the community and needs this training, local managers have not encouraged their technical training. In Rio de Janeiro, where the research was conducted, 26% of CHWs continue studying or went back to school; of these, 46% entered higher education, 17% entered high school and 24% entered technical education. Of those who entered technical education, 50% are studying nursing technician (MOTA e DAVID, 2010).

1.2.1.2 Indigenous Health Agents

The creation of the Indigenous Health Agent emerged from different movements, from the International Conference on Primary Health Care (WHO, 1978), the 1ª National Conference

of Indigenous Health Protection in 1986, arriving to the Indigenous Health Care Subsystem in 1999: the right of Indigenous peoples to participate in the planning and execution of health care in their Indigenous Lands. This position also meets many of the objectives contained in these documents, including that of being part of the health team, intermediating the knowledge of biomedical and traditional medicine, becoming the link between the community and the health team, as well as being a salaried professional (Langdon et al., 2006).

Langdon et al. (2006) add that, after the Declaration of Alma-Ata, in 1978, the goal focuses on the promotion, prevention, recovery and rehabilitation of health, which should occur at the primary level of care through health agents with a guarantee of "respect, recognition and collaboration between representatives of traditional practices and those of biomedicine. [The Declaration] recommends that traditional medicine be promoted, developed and integrated wherever possible with modern scientific medicine" (p. 2638).

The HIAs emerged in the 1980s with the important purpose of being the link between the community and the health professionals, serving as translators, since Portuguese was not spoken in many indigenous communities. However, as Novo (2010) points out, "sometimes translations are precarious, even those performed by the HIA, hindering the communication of professionals with patients and reinforcing a purely technical performance by the team" (p. 96).

Despite ideally being the fundamental "connection" between the community and the team, the HIAs, who are usually very young, do not feel able to represent the local therapeutic system, precisely because they are too young, at the same time they are little valued by the team for holding "little biomedical knowledge" (NOVO, 2010, p. 156).

Authors such as Langdon et al. (2006), Langdon and Diehl (2007), Mendonça (2005) and Garnelo et al. (2003) point out how insecure the AIS are with their actions mainly due to the ambiguity of their role: they are charged by EMSI in one way and by the indigenous community in another. Langdon et al. (2006), as well as Langdon and Diehl (2007) identified that, hierarchically in the EMSI, the AIS are forbidden to perform basic health actions, such as checking temperature, checking blood pressure and giving injections. However, the community, especially in the absence of the doctor, requires these practices, increasing the anguish of this professional in not knowing exactly how to act.

In addition to the frustration of not knowing how to define their exact functions, the ISA still needs to fill out many forms every month, which leads to more frustrations for this professional. Langdon and Diehl (2007) point out that ideally the ISA should be supervised and undergo continuous training, but, as in practice this does not occur, the forms and spreadsheets are a way of "inspecting" the ISAs' work. Adding to the bureaucratisation of the service is the eight-hour daily work routine, which raises criticism that other EMSI members work fewer hours and receive a salary that is much higher than the AIS's minimum wage (p. 25).

Both the AIS and the ACS have been included in the local systems and health services. However, in view of the pressure from the community, which demands answers through biomedicine and also from the basic care organization model itself, the agents observe the need to study more and seek knowledge through courses and diplomas recognized by western medicine.

Some studies (OLIVEIRA, 2005; MENDONÇA, 2005) show that the recognition of AISs by the team and the Health Subsystem is still lacking, and one of the alternatives would be to train the agent as a nursing assistant. In Santa Catarina, "the AISs performing or with hopes of performing Nursing Auxiliary courses perceived in this way a way to guarantee their institutional recognition and also job security" (LANGDON and DIEHL, 2007, p. 26).

1.2.2 The organisation of health care in the Xapecó Indigenous Land

In the T.I. Xapecó, during the 1970s, in addition to the mobile Funai teams, the Rural Union used to provide services in exchange for Indians who allowed non-Indian farmers to use their land. In 1978 this service was suspended after the Kaingáng expelled the farmers from their land. Until 1981, "there was only one infirmary located in the village Sede and it attended a population of 1,714 individuals", and from 1983 two other infirmaries were built, one in the village Pinhalzinho and another in the village Limeira, later expanded (NACKE et al., 2007, p. 125). At that time, three indigenous nursing attendants worked in the infirmaries, of which currently one is a nursing technician, another is an assistant and one no longer works in the health posts (more details in the chapter "The insertion of indigenous people as nursing workers").

The infirmary was considered a "mini-hospital", located in a former school, and had "a bed for occasional admissions for illnesses that required monitoring for medication, an outpatient clinic for providing first aid and preparing patients for consultations, a medical office a dental office, a medicine room, a kitchen, two bathrooms (one inoperative, attached to the bed and the other in the medical office) and a pantry-type room", besides a small room next to the medical office and a balcony, but still, it needed many reforms (DIEHL, 2001a, p. 55). From 1998, a dentist and a doctor were hired through an agreement between Funai and the municipality of Ipuaçu and started to attend twice a week in the infirmary of the village headquarters. Nursing assistants and auxiliaries were also hired through an agreement between FUNAI and a non-indigenous NGO (DIEHL, 2001a).

At that time, the most frequent diseases were respiratory infections, dehydration, scabies and measles, in addition to cases of tuberculosis, syphilis and gonorrhoea and malnutrition associated with worms, the main cause of infant mortality in the T.I. Xapecó (NACKE et al., 1983 apud HAVERROTH, 1997). The most serious or urgent cases were mainly sent to the Xanxerê hospital, as is still the case today, or to Curitiba, for the most serious cases.

Despite the efforts, the health care provided was still not sufficient. Thus, already in the new Subsystem configuration, "in January 2000, the doctor and the dentist, who had worked in the 'Infirmary' for some years, were replaced by two other professionals, who started to provide services 40 hours a week, most of the time at the village Headquarters" (DIEHL, 2001a, p. 58). In the village Pinhalzinho there was also a health post, in precarious conditions, near the highway, which had a non-indigenous nursing assistant and a doctor who attended children on Wednesday afternoons (DIEHL, 2001a).

As of 2000, health posts were installed and/or improved in the villages of Sede, Pinhalzinho, Fazenda São José and Paiol de Barro (the first three located in the territory of Ipuaçu and the last one in Entre Rios), with teams composed of at least one technician and/or nursing assistant and indigenous health agents. In the case of the larger villages such as Sede and Pinhalzinho, the team is more complete: it has a general practitioner, a gynaecologist/obstetrician, nurses, dentists, nutritionists, nursing technicians, dental assistants, indigenous health and sanitation agents, drivers and general services assistants. The professionals who work in the health posts in the part of Ipuaçu are hired by the Family Health Strategy (as is the case of the HIAs, doctor and nurse), by the agreement between the NGO Associação Rondon and FUNASA (doctor, nurses, dentist, nutritionist, nursing technicians and assistants, dental office assistants, indigenous sanitation agents) and also by FUNASA as federal public servants (one technician and one nursing assistant). In Entre Rios, the professionals are hired through an agreement between the municipal government and the NGO Rondon Brazil.

The members of the non-indigenous health teams live mostly in Xanxerê and travel daily to the health posts in the T.I. Xapecó. Most of the time they travel in Funasa cars. They remain in the village from 8am to 5pm[11] and have lunch at the health post itself, which has a kitchen equipped with a refrigerator, cooker and table.

The EMSI send monthly reports, called consolidated reports, to the local coordination, located in Chapecó, SC. The purpose of these consolidated reports is to feed the Indigenous Health Information System (SIASI).

The Xapecó Indigenous Lands form part of the Southern Interior SDI (Figure 7), which also covers the states of São Paulo, Paraná and Rio Grande do Sul in its western portions.

Since the establishment of the DSEI Interior Sul, it is clear that the services have been better structured, both through the presence of the EMSI and more physical infrastructure, with the construction of health posts. The demands continue to be infectious and parasitic diseases, with the addition of chronic degenerative diseases, such as diabetes, cardiovascular diseases (including hypertension) and cancer.

1.3 Nursing and indigenous health

1.3.1 Nursing care

Nursing is caring. This is the essence of every nurse - caring. According to Waldow et al. (1995), it is from the 1980s onwards that reflections on caring and how care is provided began. The questions of how to provide care, who should do it, and how arose. It is at this time that questions such as the value of care and caring begin to emerge. It is also in this period that the question of to whom the practice of caring belongs and where it should start from: patients, schools, or nursing itself.

Patient care has a long history and has undergone many changes throughout history and the notions of caring and care, which have been changing. However, despite the changes in the concepts of caring and care, care remains the premise of nursing - caring. Among the nursing theorists who discuss and study the forms of care, Madeleine M. Leininger, who, in the 1950s and working with children from different ethnic groups, observed that they had different care needs, developed her transcultural theory of care:

> *What the people need most to grow, remain well, avoid illness and survive or to face death is human caring; Care is the essence of nursing and the distinct, dominant, central, and unifying, focus of nursing; Caring is the "heart and soul" of nursing and what people seek most from professional nurses and in health care services; Nurses are therefore challenged to gain knowledge to care for well and sick people; Cultural Care theory and use of research findings from many different cultures constitutes the new challenge for nurses in providing meaningful and congruent care to people of the world[1]* (LEININGER, 1991, p. 5. 5).

Leininger realised that, in addition to the universal care of birth, growth and death, there were different forms of local behaviour and care, and it seemed that these patterns were related to cultural issues. She sought subsidies to understand this differentiation of caring and care in anthropology and concluded that this knowledge was extremely important for nursing. For three decades she studied and published an extensive and intense work (WALDOW et al., 1995).

This is a challenging job, since nursing is based on the positivist model of medicine, centered on cure and disease. Efficient nursing that knows technical terms recognises signs and symptoms and knows how to "read" exams and diagnoses in their care is still highly valued. Leininger observes this emphasis on technical care and is concerned with the "humanizing" of this care, as he did not find, among the theories already written, rooted in positivist logic, one that suited his needs for understanding care in its various dimensions. (WALDOW et al., 1995)

Based on anthropology, Leininger develops his own nursing research model, called ethnoenfer nursing, in which the prefix *ethno* refers to people from the community, ideas and cultural practices with regard to nursing care. This method was developed to help nurses understand, through observation, the meaning of these everyday experiences with regard to care in any context. As time went by, Leininger refined his method and turned more to the *emic* side, that is, of perceptions internal to the group, rather than *ethic,* that is, "outside" the group studied. Initially, this type of research was not considered scientific, since at that time only statistical data was valued (WALDOW et al., 1995, p. 12).

According to Leininger, our world changes very quickly, and the multicultural growth is a transforming reality to which nursing should be attentive to better understand and assist individuals in their most vulnerable moments, respecting the differences of understanding about health, disease, care, well-being, and death. The theory of Cultural Care encourages nurses to study and understand the different ways of perceiving these factors to better serve their client/patient, because without this understanding there will be no comprehension on both sides of the care to be provided, generating great frustration, confusion and anger, at which point the theory gains relevance in helping to understand the differences (LEININGER, 1991).

In his theory there are three modalities to guide nurses in their judgements, decisions and actions: 1) cultural preservation and/or maintenance care; 2) accommodation to cultural care and/or negotiation; 3) the repatterning or restructuring of cultural care (LEININGER, 1991, p. 40).

However, 'accommodation' is the opposite of 'negotiation', because while accommodation suggests something passive, negotiation involves a conversation to reach a common point (BOEHS, 2002).

Nursing needs anthropology to understand that there are differences, and that these differences do not necessarily make things worse or better: they are just different, but it will be necessary to find a congruent point between the caregiver and the being cared for, aiming at the patient's well-being. As Boehs (2002) puts it, it is a great theory, but it is necessary to rethink how to put it into practice: "There are questions, how to take into account cultural factors using principles of non-intervention anthropology, but at the same time, being a nursing professional who is a profession whose principle is to intervene" (p. 91).

Leininger's theory does not provide a "formula" on how to care for the patient while respecting his/her diversity and simultaneously providing technical care, but rather a concern with the need to "dialogue, spend more time with the client, provide support, be present to the needs, trust, respect, provide opportunities and take into account, understand, and listen. In the transcultural nursing literature, Leininger and his followers hope to achieve congruence of care between the explanatory model of the client/family and the professional" (BOEHS, 2002, p. 94).

Nursing is a profession that is dedicated to caring for others. Caring for the other implies knowing and respecting him/her. It does not mean that, by knowing him/her, the actions will become easier; they will at least become respectful to the caregiver and the cared-for, creating a bond of mutual respect. Boehs (2002) emphasizes that:

> The great challenge for nurses who venture into the paths of anthropology to care for the human being in a more comprehensive way is certainly to perform the anthropological look. That is, within the nursing culture, to take off for a moment the armour of the professional model and see the client in his world, understand his actions, but at the same time not ceasing to be the nurse. How to be one and the other at the same time? Leininger's theory is a proposal to overcome this challenge. However, as it is a comprehensive

theory, it has abstract concepts, thus there is a wide field to give more answers to the challenge of how to use this anthropological vision in nursing. In Brazil, Leininger's theory has brought nurses closer and closer to anthropology. Undoubtedly, using a theory based on anthropology and nursing is a contribution to bring the world of the client closer to the world of the health professional and to foster knowledge in nursing. For this to occur, we must be careful not to apply the theory in a repetitive manner, without critical evaluations, running the risk of wasting energy in vain. Leininger's theory, as well as other approaches based on anthropology, has limitations, and, as shown in the analysis of this paper, has ambiguities, terms that need to be clarified within the context where they will be applied (p. 95).

1.3.2 Nursing technicians and auxiliaries and caring

Nursing qualification and its activities differ worldwide, since nursing practice is influenced by the political, economic and cultural reality surrounding it. This care is individual, family, community and includes health promotion, disease prevention, treatment of patients with chronic or acute diseases, patients in rehabilitation or even monitoring of terminally ill patients (ROCHA and ALMEIDA, 2000, p. 97).

Mid-level nursing professionals, auxiliary and technical, have different backgrounds, but as will be seen in the chapter "Activities performed by nursing auxiliaries and technicians", in the exercise of their functions, however, in primary care practice both exercise practically the same activities.

According to Shimizu et al. (2004), the work of nursing technicians and assistants highlights the care provided to spontaneous demand. They are also the ones who perform triage and verify the need for referral when there is no doctor present in health care. The working conditions of the family health teams are still precarious, and many times, due to the lack of human resources, mid-level professionals work without direct supervision, being necessary to take on responsibilities beyond their professional duties. Also according to these authors, much of the work of family health teams depends on the work of nursing assistants, which makes training for these professionals necessary and urgent.

Crossetti et al. (2000), in their study on caring from the perspective of students in a professional training course, identified that care is perceived in two ways: expressive care and professional care. The elements of expressive care are: affection, giving of oneself, presence, protection, concern, availability, understanding, respect, comfort, responsibility, solidarity, safety, intentionality, sharing/exchange. On the other hand, the elements of professional care expressed by the study subjects are: assisting/caregiving, technical competence, professional knowledge and liking what they do (p. 67). The authors observed that middle-level professionals value expressive care much more than professional care. This reflects a quality in the training of these professionals, and, consequently, an appreciation of the care provided to their future patients/clients.

Although the health model has advanced, emphasizing care over the family and the community, some nursing professionals are still concerned with biologicist, technological care, centered on disease and procedures. This occurs because nursing is initially sought as a profession to "help people". However, its "fragility" is perceived as it is not considered "scientific", and, therefore, the legitimisation of this profession is sought in technical procedures, as Wendhausen and Rivera (2005) put it:

> When we resume the reasons for our professional choice in nursing, we find that many of them, such as "wanting to do something for people", "liking people", "liking to care for people", "wanting to help", etc., are related to the human aspects of caring, often considered less valuable by many professionals. Therefore, in this rescue of our humanity, it is necessary to re-signify them, valuing them as internal mobilization of what is human in us (p. 112).

It is noticeable that the reasons that led the professional to the nursing course are contradictory to their actions due to the need to "scientificify" their procedures. As will be seen in the chapter "The insertion of indigenous people as nursing workers", the motivation to enter nursing is to help, to care for the other. However, the courses are focused on the technical production of knowledge, as mentioned above, and the care model performed by these professionals is technicist and uncritical reproduction of existing practices (RIBEIRO and PEDRÃO, 2005).

The Family Health Strategy (ESF), created in 1994 by the Ministry of Health, as the Family Health Programme (PSF), was a strategy for the reorientation of the care model from the organisation of primary care, focusing on the "establishment of links and [on] the creation of bonds of commitment and co-responsibility between health professionals and the population" (BRASIL, 1997, p. 7). Among these professionals are the technicians and nursing assistants.

Schimith et al. (2004) state that the PSF aims to bring the health team closer to the user, creating a link in order to provide a welcoming assistance:

> The program does not refer to the bond with the possibility of autonomy of the user, nor with their participation in the organization of the service. The link should be extensive to the entire health team, because only in this way is it possible to actually meet the demands and needs of the real subjects of

health work. It is necessary that the welcoming and bonding project be a project of the entire team, so that it is materialized in the live work in act. For this to occur, the nurse should make his work more focused on the clinic, valuing the reception and the bond with the service user and becoming a professional with greater resolutivity (p. 1491).

CHAPTER 2

2 Trajectory and methodology

2.1 Trajectory

To begin this work, it is necessary to locate it in my trajectory until the present moment. I am a nurse who graduated from the Federal University of Paraná (UFPR) in 1999. I worked as a nurse in the Family Health Program, currently the Family Health Strategy, but I was also an administrative nurse in a small hospital in the interior of Paraná. I worked in technical education as a teacher and later as a pedagogical coordinator for the Project for Professionalization of Nursing Workers (Profae) from 2001 to 2005. In this period, I attended a specialization course in Pedagogy of Technical Education at the Oswaldo Cruz Foundation promoted by PROFAE. Afterwards (2002), I worked at the State Secretary of Health of Paraná evaluating technical courses in the health area, when I then sent my curriculum to the North of the country, to work with indigenous health.

I started working in indigenous health in 2006, first in Pará, as technical coordinator, and then in Amazonas, as a care nurse, totaling two years of work. During this period working with indigenous health, it was possible to get to know and work with the Munduruku, Kaiapó, Mura, Apurinã, Sateré-Mawé, Baré, Tukano, and Tikuna ethnic groups, among others. When I worked as a nurse in these different communities and ethnicities, it was possible to experience the cultural differences[13] existing between the various indigenous villages. This period was very distressing for me, as it was at odds with the mission of the employing body with the activities developed. In addition to this fact, in the various meetings and gatherings between employees who worked with indigenous health, comments were common regarding the way of life of the indigenous people and their culpability for their illnesses and eventual deaths.

Many questions troubled me in this period: on the one hand, I heard that "health professionals should be transforming agents, to help them understand what hygiene is and how to prevent diseases", and on the other I received information that "we should not change their habits and customs and culture should be respected". How to act in the face of conflicting statements?

Thus, on returning to the South, I had the opportunity to attend a seminar on indigenous health at the UFPR, where Dr Esther Jean Langdon spoke about research being carried out on indigenous health. Her eloquence in speaking was the decisive factor for me to seek her out in Florianópolis in search of guidance for my Masters degree. But anthropology was (and is?) very distant from my understanding. Thus, associating public health and anthropology, is that this work was born, under the guidance of Professor Eliana Diehl.

The search for the understanding of anthropology begins in this period, but it is not easy. Due to my biomedical training, it becomes complex to undress the pre-formed concepts to embark on the path of anthropology, which presupposes understanding the perspective of the other, including their knowledge, experiences and practices.

Anthropology showed me that the concept of culture - still perceived this way by many colleagues in health - is not shown as I conceived it previously, i.e., as fixed actions and perceptions that do not change. On the contrary, Geertz (1978) shows that culture is a network of symbols, and that "the man is an animal entangled in webs of meanings which he himself has woven" (GEERTZ, 1978, p. 15). Thus, "culture" is not something static, but are behaviours, thoughts, meanings that are constantly changing and in interaction with the other, emerging from the context, i.e., it is not defined *a priori*.

So, after defining that we would develop a research on indigenous health in the collective health approach with an approximation to anthropology, we needed to delimit the field of work. Considering that various studies on indigenous health agents have been conducted in the country and that the training of indigenous people in health professions has been observed, we decided on the theme of indigenous nursing technicians and assistants, selecting the Kaingáng ethnic group of the Xapecó Indigenous Land.

Firstly, the cacique of the T.I. Xapecó was contacted in January 2010 to request permission to carry out the research, which was granted in February of the same year. With this document, the legal processing of the project began (ethical opinion and authorisation to enter an Indigenous Land). This research was submitted to the public notice of the National Research Institute Brasil Plural and approved funding for the fieldwork, which totalled 60 days in the T.I. Xapecó between the months of December 2010 and January and February 2011. In August 2010, together with my supervisor, I went to visit the Indigenous Land and establish the first contacts, including the verification of the possibility of housing.

I stayed a few days in November 2010 in the city of Ipuaçu and the village Sede, which served to request permission from the cacique elected after approval of the project and, so to speak, "break the ice" of my entry into the area.

I went effectively for the field research on the first days of January, but the resident of the house where I would stay was travelling to take care of her health, which led me to stay for two nights in the city of Xanxerê, 32 km from the village Sede. This was a complicating factor in the first two days. However, after my introduction, my host's family invited me to stay with them, facilitating my immersion in the village.

I stayed with this family until the return of my host, who hosted me for almost the entire period of my stay. Initially, the intention was to stay for about a week in each village to be researched, in different houses, to get different points of view. However, some problems made this mobility impossible: among them, the rain and the lack of a car. The first problem makes it difficult to get to some parts of the Indigenous Land, and the second makes it difficult to cover distances of almost 50 km inside the villages.

In the month of January I stayed in the health post of the main village, the village Sede, during all their working hours. I introduced myself to the health team and asked every day for permission to "follow" them in their daily activities. I would accompany the assistants and technicians in their routine consultations, writing down in my field diary what was said and done. When possible, I questioned the residents about their activities and actions and, if possible, I even interviewed them. At nights and weekends I socialized with the family where I stayed, visiting their friends, participating in festive gatherings, dinners at the homes of others and going to the evangelical church my hostess attended.

On the last Sunday in January, after we had celebrated the birthday of the youngest member of the family that was hosting me, a dispute between groups for the "cacicado" began in the Sede village, making the context not very propitious for field research. So I left the T.I. Xapecó, returning a week later when the "moods" were calmer. I returned with my own car, which gave me more mobility to go to the villages that still remained to be researched. So for almost two weeks, on alternate days, my host and I would go to the village Pinhalzinho - I to do research, and she to visit family. I would stay during office hours at the health post in this village and we would return in the afternoon to my host's house in the village Sede. There were two visits to the village Fazenda São José, but due to the rains the doctor had not made his fortnightly visits since the beginning of the year, so the activities were reduced.

In the Paiol de Barro village I stayed two days and one night. I was invited by the indigenous nursing technician to stay overnight in her home. Thus, I could observe her in her work of preparing the multimixture (a preparation of various cereals, among other foods, taught by the Health Pastoral and the Children's Pastoral, both of the Catholic Church), herbal soap and syrups, as well as in her care and guidance to the community. In this village I also attended a meeting with the indigenous health agents on their first day of work after being approved in the municipal selection process.

The period in the field had many interferences, such as the dismissal and rehiring of indigenous health agents, the holiday of various professionals, two internal disputes over the position of chief and various interferences in health care due to the transition from the National Health Foundation to the Special Indigenous Health Secretariat (Sesai).

Thus, in the period of a little over two months, including the first visit in August 2010, it was possible to follow and visualise the work of medium-level indigenous professionals in their communities, using the ethnographic method.

2.1 Methodology

The present study, of a descriptive qualitative nature, sought to identify and monitor the nursing auxiliaries and technicians of the T.I. Xapecó, Santa Catarina.

Data were collected through two main strategies: secondary research (documentary/bibliographical) referring to the courses for training nursing technicians/auxiliaries and field research based on qualitative anthropological methods, that is, ethnographic research.

2.1.1 Secondary research

The bibliographic research was carried out in the SciELO, LILACS and Capes Theses databases, using the keywords "técnico ou auxiliar de enfermagem", "profissionais indígenas de saúde", "agentes indígenas de saúde" and "Profae" as keywords. In addition, books and other publications, as in electronic sites, were also consulted.

The research on documents provided for all and any documentation related to the mid-level training courses in health carried out by indigenous people, such as handouts, political-pedagogical projects, certificates, among others, as well as the legislation surrounding this training. Access to the documents on the mid-level professional training course for indigenous people offered by the Federal University of Santa Catarina (UFSC) was denied us by the coordination, just as there was no access to the documents of the other courses due to the impossibility of contacting the respective coordinations (there was no response on their part). Thus, the documental analysis was based on documents collected from the indigenous professionals of the T.I. Xapecó. The documentary research was complemented by an interview with a teacher from the course at the UFSC.

2.1.2 Ethnographic research

The ethnographic method presents itself as a specific form of constructing a narrative about the social group researched. To this end, a field research was conducted for two months with the aim of observing the nursing practices performed by mid-level professionals, as well as interviewing the nursing assistants and technicians.

Ethnography, according to Geertz (1978), "is about establishing relationships, selecting informants, transcribing texts, raising genealogies, mapping fields, keeping a diary, and so on" (p. 15).

Ethnography is not only an observational activity, but also an interpretative one, not just about collecting data, but about "decoding" it:

There are three characteristics of ethnographic description: it

> is interpretative; what it interprets is the flow of social discourse and the interpretation involved consists in saving the 'said' in such discourse from its possibility of becoming extinct and fixing it in researchable forms (GEERTZ, 1978, p. 31).

Thus, the techniques of interviews (semi-structured and open) and participant observation were used. For the interviews (see scripts in Appendices 1, 2 and 3), the interviewee was instructed about the research according to the Free and Informed Consent Form (Appendices 4, 5 and 6), which was signed when there was agreement to participate. The members of the Multidisciplinary Teams for Basic Indigenous Health Care (EMSI) were interviewed about the role of indigenous nursing technicians and assistants, emphasizing the self-perception and perception of this role.

The activities of nursing technicians and auxiliaries (indigenous and non-indigenous) and the rest of the EMSI in the health posts of the villages Sede, Pinhalzinho, Fazenda São José and Paiol de Barro were observed and followed.

The subjects of this research were, therefore, the teacher of the course for training of nursing technicians/auxiliaries (UFSC), the EMSI professionals, especially the nursing technicians/auxiliaries (indigenous and non-indigenous) and eventually some users of health care services.

For data recording, the field diary and voice recording were used, in addition to photographic registration. The analysis of qualitative data focused on the identification of symbolic meanings emerging within the interviews and on participant observation, i.e., in the common aspects of the players involved in their speeches on the same subject, themes and issues, allowing the systematization of convergent points. The points of divergence were analysed from the context of speech and of who speaks, paying attention to the place and situation in which the conversation/interview was held, as well as the location of the interlocutor in a given network of social relations. In short, the analytical effort proposed to qualitatively evaluate the care provided in health actions and services from the point of view of the actors involved. The data on the profile of the EMSI and the sociodemographic profile of indigenous nursing technicians and assistants were analyzed according to their frequency.

2.1.3   Study location and research subjects

The Xapecó Indigenous Land was selected with reference to the villages Sede, Pinhalzinho and Fazenda São José (geographically located in the municipality of Ipuaçu) and the village Paiol de Barro (located in the municipality of Entre Rios), mainly because for the past 17 years the research group coordinated by Professors Esther Jean Langdon and Eliana E. Diehl has been developing research among the Kaingáng, with established links that facilitate access to information and the collection of data. The T.I. Xapecó is inhabited mainly by the Kaingáng (about 4,000 inhabitants), a Jê group that is found from São Paulo to Rio Grande do Sul and is the second largest group in the country. The Kaingáng speak Portuguese and have a long history of contact with non-Indians. Further details have already been described in the literature review.

The field research was conducted over 60 days (December 2010 to February 2011) in the villages Sede, Pinhalzinho and Fazenda São José (geographically located in the municipality of Ipuaçu) and in the village Paiol de Barro (located in the municipality of Entre Rios), where there are health posts. The monitoring of the professionals' work occurred in the health posts of the village Sede, the main village, the village Pinhalzinho, the village Paiol de Barro and two visits to the village Fazenda São José.

The subjects were a teacher of the course for training nursing technicians/auxiliaries (UFSC), a coordinator of the 1994 Course, the EMSI professionals, especially the nursing technicians/auxiliaries (indigenous and non-indigenous) and eventually some users of health care services, totalling 16 people. The coordinator of one of the courses refused to participate in the research and it was not possible to contact the other teachers and coordinators.

Members of the EMSI were interviewed about the perception of the role of indigenous nursing technicians and auxiliaries. The activities of nursing technicians and auxiliaries and the rest of the EMSI in the health posts were observed and monitored. All the interviewees signed the Informed Consent Form. In addition, the activities of nursing technicians and auxiliaries (indigenous and non-indigenous) and the rest of the MRESI in the health posts were observed and monitored. For reasons of confidentiality and anonymity, all names have been changed.

2.1.4   Data recording and analysis

For data recording, the field diary and voice recording (whenever allowed) were used, in addition to photographic record. The analysis of qualitative data focused on the identification of symbolic meanings emerging within the interviews and participant observation, i.e., in the common aspects of the players involved in their speeches on the same subject, themes and issues, allowing the systematization of convergent points. The points of divergence were analysed from the context of speech and of who speaks, paying attention to the place and situation in which the conversation/interview was held, as well as the location of the interlocutor in a given network of social relations. In short, the analytical effort proposed to qualitatively evaluate the attention performed in health actions and services from the points of view of the actors involved. The data on the profile of the EMSI and the sociodemographic profile of indigenous nursing technicians and assistants were analyzed according to their frequency.

2.1.5 Ethical aspects

This research complied with Resolution 196/CNS/1996, receiving Opinion no.º 626/2010 from the UFSC Ethics Committee for Research with Human Beings (Appendix 1) and Opinion no.º 40/2010 (Registration no.º 16034) from the National Commission for Ethics in Research (Conep) (Appendix 2). He received the Authorization for Entry into Indigenous Land nº 90/AAEP/2010 from the National Indian Foundation (Funai) (Attachment 3).

CHAPTER 3

3 The insertion of indigenous people as nursing workers

3.1 Profile of health professionals: nursing auxiliaries and technicians

In the context of indigenous health, a gradual increase in the number of indigenous people seeking training and working as Nursing technicians or assistants is observed. Considering the entire I.T. Xapecó, between December 2010 and February 2011, the two EMSI were composed of professionals as shown in Table 1. It should be noted that, as usually happens during this period of the year, many professionals had been dismissed due to the end of their contract and were awaiting a new selection process, such as the AIS and the physician in the Entre Rios area.

Table 2 shows the number of EMSI members in 2004, according to Langdon et al. (2006). It is possible to note that there were no nursing technicians in this period, but nine nursing assistants. In 2011, this number increased to eight technicians and three nursing assistants (Table 1). Also in 2011, the number of nurses and dental assistants increased and a nutritionist was added to the current team.

In the T.I. Xapecó there were a total of 17 medium-level nursing professionals (among those who were working and unemployed). Three were nursing assistants; the others were technicians, all graduated through free professionalizing courses; one of the technicians is not indigenous (Table 2).

One of the reasons for unemployment involves internal political alliances, similar to what was observed among the AIS (for details, see LANGDON et al., 2006), that is, technicians/auxiliaries that have no connection with the leadership have less chance of being employed. The reason why the residents do not go out in search of work outside of the Indigenous Land, as reported by themselves or the community, is the distance from their families, as they do not accept the idea of being far from their relatives and friends.

Table 1 - Profile of the EMSI, Xapecó Indigenous Land, SC, Dec. 2010/Feb. 2011.

EMSI Professional	Fem. (n)°	Male (n)°
Indigenous Health Agent	15	2
Indigenous Sanitation Agent	0	2
Indigenous Nursing Technician	2	5
Indigenous Nursing Auxiliary	2	1
Non-indigenous Nursing Technician	1	0
Non-indigenous Nursing Auxiliary	0	0
Dental Office Assistant	2	0
Nurse	6	0
Dentist	1	1
Nutritionist	1	0
Doctor	0	2

Table 2 - Health professionals in the Xapecó Indigenous Land, May - July, 2004.

EMSI Professional	N°
Indigenous Health Agent	21
Indigenous Sanitation Agent	5
Nursing Technician	-
Nursing Auxiliary	9
Dental Office Assistant	1
Nurse	3
Dentist	2
Nutritionist	-
Doctor	2

Source: adapted from Langdon et al. (2006, p. 2041).

Among the 16 indigenous people, the majority was aged between 31 and 50 years and they are equally divided between men and women. Among those who informed, most were married or lived together with their partner, had up to three children and were Kaingáng, although they did not speak the language (Table 2). Three technicians had higher education, one of whom worked as a nursing technician, one had always worked in the administration of the agreement between the NGO and FUNASA, and another was studying for higher education.

In general, they are eager for more capacity building and training, which demonstrates their desire to continue updating:

> In fact, I had a dream of becoming a nurse, I still have one, and that's why I got the job as an auxiliary nurse at the time of the late Ourides. Most of them were from the head office, but my dream was to become a nurse. But as my salary, and having to leave my job to study, it is not possible to go to college, it is very difficult, but it is a dream. I always got on well with the health team, but we have a problem that changes a lot, not the technicians, but the nurses who come from outside. Because it always involves politics, and we've always had problems with agreements. I would have the opportunity to take the [public] exam and go to the city [Entre Rios], because here every contract is difficult, and my husband is in politics, but I didn't want to do it because I like it here, the work and they also like my work (Techn. Ind. Enf Amanda).

There are ten indigenous professionals working in functions compatible with their training, however, there is one technician working as an AIS and another in general services, with the majority receiving between R$701.00 and R$1,000.00. When questioned about working in other functions, the response of the professional who works in general services was:

> We don't know what will happen tomorrow, there is a lot of insecurity in our work. Because I moved from Funasa to the Secretariat this year, there is a lot of insecurity among the employees about what is going to happen. I preferred to stay as a general service because I have more stability and the mayor even gave me a raise because I have a technical course (Aux. Serv. Gerais Luana).

Table 2 - Profile of indigenous nursing technicians/assistants, Xapecó Indigenous Land, SC, Dec. 2010/Feb. 2011.

Sex	Female	8
	Male	8
Age Group	Between 21 and 30 years old	2
	Between 31 and 40 years old	8
	Between 41 and 50 years old	3
	Over 51 years old	3
Schooling	Elementary School complete	1
	High School complete	12
	Higher Education Complete	3
Civil status	Married/Living together	8
	Widower	1
	Separated	1
	Not informed	6
Number of children	no	1
	an	3
	two	5
	three or more	1
	Not informed	6
Ethnicity	Kaingáng	6
	Xeta	1
	Kaingáng-Guarani	1
	Not informed	8
Indigenous language	Does not understand and does not speak	6
	Understands but does not speak	2
	Understands and speaks	2
	Not informed	6
Acting	Currently working in	

professional		10
	function compatible with training Contracted for other Activities	2
	Unemployed	4
Income monthly (R$)	510,00 - 700,00	1
	701,00 - 1.000,00	8
	1.001,00 - 1.500,00	1
	Not informed	2

The instability of employment that normally occurs at the end and beginning of the year due to the expiry of the contracts of the professionals and the changes in the organisation of indigenous health, with FUNASA's administration passing to the Special Secretariat of Indigenous Health (SESAI), cause insecurity and much distress among the professionals and the community. According to Article 6 of Decree n° 7.336/2010, altered by Decree n° 7.461/2011: "The Ministry of Health and the National Health Foundation should effect the transition of the management of the Indigenous Health Care Subsystem to the Ministry of Health by 31 December 2011" (BRASIL, 2011c, p. 1).

Until the time of my fieldwork (end of February 2011), the transition between FUNASA and SESAI was a cause of great concern in the indigenous community, because specialist consultations, exams, purchases and payments by the agreement administrator had been suspended in order to await the end of the transition, which, according to Decree no.° 7.336/2010, should occur within 180 days from October. However, the alteration of the Decree changed the transition deadline to December 31, 2011, maintaining the current organizational structure. With this, salary payments, fuel supply, special medicines and specialist consultations were delayed, with no date to be regulated.

3.2 Training of nursing auxiliaries and technicians at T.I. Xapecó

Some of the medium level indigenous professionals working in the T.I. Xapecó completed their courses through institutions that had the objective of professionalising workers who were already working in the health area.

Among the 13 indigenous nursing technicians, ten started and concluded a course promoted by the Federal University of Santa Catarina, called "Projeto Pioneiro". The "Pioneer Project" was composed of two phases: nursing auxiliary, in the years 2002 and 2003, and nursing technician, between 2004 and 2005. Eight students who completed the auxiliary course through this project also finished the technical course, with the addition of two more Indians who had completed the auxiliary course through other institutions (Table 3).

The three indigenous nursing assistants working during this research completed free courses through different institutions, namely: Professionalization Project for Workers in the Nursing Area (Profae) at the National Commercial Learning Service (Senac), in 2003 (two indigenous people); and Nursing Assistant Professional Qualification Supletive Course, in 1994, Braga, RS.

It is important to highlight that two of the indigenous professionals who exercised the function of nursing attendants at the time of the Funai have recycled their knowledge in the recent courses cited in Table 3. These two professionals had taken a free correspondence course at the Rio Branco Institute to train as attendants between January and June 1988. Currently, one of them is a nursing assistant and the other a nursing technician. Another professional took the course of hospital attendant by the Ministry of Social Welfare and Assistance from April to May 1978, and today she is a nursing technician, but works in another function. These professionals have been working for many years in T.I. Xapecó, as one of them says:

> I did the first attendant course by correspondence approximately 30 years ago, it was not valid, but it gave you a notion (...). At that time you did the nursing attendant to teach you how to do sutures, deliveries, you did everything, not today, but at that time it was. The attendant was the doctor, in that countryside there (Technician Ind. Nurse Carlos).

Table 3 - Professional courses taken by indigenous people, Xapecó Indigenous Land, SC.

Training	Nursing auxiliary	Nursing technician
Supplementary Professional Qualification Course for Nursing Auxiliary (1994)	4	-
Senac/Profae, Nursing Assistant (2003)	3	-
Health Training School (Profae), Nursing Technician (2004)	-	4

| Nursing auxiliary course (UFSC) (2002/2003) | 8 | - |
| Nursing Technician Course (UFSC) (2004/2005) | - | 10 |

In the T.I. Xapecó there are three indigenous nursing technicians who have already worked as indigenous health agents (AIS) and one technician who still works as an AIS.

Among the courses offered, it was observed that one of them (promoted by the UFSC) offered a course focused on aspects of the region of the Xapecó Indigenous Territory and its customs, but none of them specifically considered the sociocultural, political and economic context of the Kaingáng. According to Castro (2007), there are doubts whether one should organize courses directed only to the Indians, even if this is the ideal, as was the case of the "Projeto Xamã" (Shaman Project) of the Bakairi Indians, Mato Grosso, who claimed a training to legitimize their performance. This author points out that as the project was specifically aimed at indigenous people of a region of Mato Grosso, they did not attend the traditional nursing assistant course, with hospital internship, leading the indigenous professionals of the health teams to question their training. These indigenous nursing auxiliaries felt less capable than the nursing auxiliaries who did their training with hospital internship.

3.2.1 Supplementary professional qualification course for nursing auxiliaries, 1994

The first course to be offered specifically for the indigenous population began in 1993, promoted by the Immaculate Heart of Mary Sisterhood of the Catholic Church, together with the Lutheran Church and the Indigenous Missionary Council (CIMI). The course lasted one month of theoretical classes in Braga (RS) and one month of practical classes in the villages at the students' homes. According to the religious Sara, 13 vacancies were requested for the Kaingáng, but some conditions were imposed: the vacancies should be distributed among other ethnic groups, and Sister Sara should accompany the internships of the indigenous participants. For this sister, there was the understanding that the training of indigenous people would provide better service in the villages:

Most of the nursing technicians on indigenous land were white

people who didn't understand Indian culture. And the
indigenous nursing technician knew the community, the teas,
the culture and knew the people better (...). The indigenous
nursing technician accompanies the patients more. He knows
the community to work with the medicines right at home
(Sister Sara).

This course had as its central issue the teaching of medicinal plants, since some of the sisters of the Congregation understood that:

> The course was with the rescue of traditional indigenous
> medicine, respect for their culture, differentiated treatment in
> hospitals. This was because it was important to understand the
> need to accompany the indigenous people, especially those
> who did not speak Portuguese (Sister Sara).

The emphasis on medicinal plants contemplated at least two objectives. The first of these, which is not explicit, concerns the form of action of the Pastoral da Saúde, that is, encouraging the use of such resources

therapeutic by any social groups and communities, whether urban or rural. The second objective was explicitly related to the "rescue of traditional medicine" as part of indigenous culture, as pointed out by Sister Sara:

> It is necessary to know the culture well to have this respect,
> the question of teas, of roots, of blessings. Respecting this (...).
> The cultivation of plants was also being lost, and the culture
> of planting for their own consumption and for their own
> sustenance was also being lost (Sister Sara).

Also according to the sister, for many years the use of plants was prevented in the Indigenous Lands in the South of the country, which demonstrated the importance of such a "rescue": "FUNAI did not allow the working of the teas, they only allowed ready-made medicine to treat sick Indians" (Sister Sara).

According to this sister, involved in the project at the time, there were 480 hours of internship in hospitals and health posts, with one month of theoretical classes in Braga, RS, and one month of practice in the villages of each ethnic group, totalling 1,300 hours of training.

> The old ones came to help in the teaching of the teas, of the
> remedies (about the course, where the old healers, healers,
> shamans, were called to give lessons and explanations of the
> plants and teas) (Sister Sara).

Of the four indigenous people who graduated from this course, two took the technical course promoted by the UFSC, one became a technician through PROFAE and the fourth remains as an auxiliary.

3.2.2 Project for the professionalization of nursing workers (Profae), 2003 and 2004

The Professionalization of Nursing Workers Project emerged on 15 October 1999, through Ordinance n° 1.262/GM[14] , with the aim of training and certifying professionals who

were active in health in the area of nursing, but did not have training consistent with the activities performed. The milestone was in 2000, with the first class in the state of Espírito Santo.

It was estimated that in 1999, there were 250 thousand professionals, at that time called medium level, but they were nursing assistants, without the necessary qualification and knowledge for their practices. The amount of professionals working was significant, and many had started working in hospitals and health posts without minimum education: they were people of low income, which made it difficult to access the private professionalizing courses that existed in the country (BRASIL, 2003).

The Project started with a partnership between the Ministry of Labour and the Ministry of Health, managed by the latter, and its actions were decentralized in the states and municipalities where the courses were executed by private entities, through bidding, and mainly in public Technical Schools. Among its objectives, we can highlight:

> PROFAE also seeks to strengthen the institutions that work with Human Resources in the area of health, providing technical and financial support for professional qualification and education. Among the actions aimed at institutional strengthening are the Pedagogical Training Course for the specialisation of Nurses; the Modernisation and Creation of Technical Health Schools of the SUS; the elaboration and implementation of a Professional Skills Certification System; and the implementation of an Information System on the Labour Market in Health, with a focus on Nursing (BRASIL, 2003).

Currently, PROFAE courses are offered exclusively by SUS Technical Schools. There are a total of 36 schools, 33 state, two municipal, and one federal, focused on the training of middle-level workers in the health system, belonging to the Network of Technical Schools of the SUS/RET-SUS. This network brings together the Ministry of Health, the National Council of Health Secretaries

(CONASS) and the National Council of Municipal Health Secretaries (Conasems) (BRASIL, 2011d).Profae proposes an innovative methodology: through the problematization technique, it uses the "arc of Maguerez" (Figure 9). This methodology aims to bring everyday work problems to the classroom, where they share their understanding of the problems and their possible solutions.

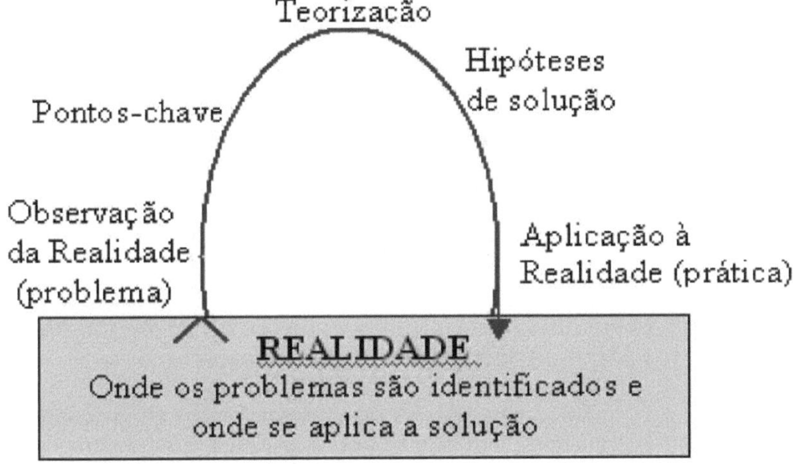

Figure 8 - Maguerez's Arc. Available at: <http://www.abed.org.br/ congress2004/by/htm/112-TC-D1.htmA>.

The course is divided into two modules. The first module is the Technical Qualification - Nursing Assistant of the Nursing Technical Course, lasting 1,250 hours, of which 400 hours are internship. The second module is the Qualification in Nursing Technician, lasting 1,800 hours, of which 600 hours are supervised internship.

Among the three indigenous auxiliaries trained by Profae, two remain with this training and are hired as nursing auxiliaries and one did the nursing technician by the "Pioneer Project".

The three technicians certified by Profae are hired and work according to their training, although one of the technicians has attended college.

3.2.3 The "Pioneer Project" (UFSC)

Initially, the "Projeto Pioneiro" was not specifically intended to train indigenous people. It was created by the Government of the State of Santa Catarina, within a macroproject financed by the Ministry of Labour in agreement with the UFSC, for the training of nursing auxiliaries and technicians.

The Federal University of Santa Catarina had its involvement with this project through the Nursing Graduate Network of the Southern Region

(REPENSUL) and the Undergraduate Nursing School, in addition to the participation of the Regional Councils of Nursing of the southern region. This trajectory began with the training of masters and doctors for the Federal Universities of Paraná, Santa Catarina and Rio Grande do Sul. Later, this model of work was extended to the training of middle level professionals, when it was financed by the Ministry of Labor.

The project was considered pioneering because the pedagogical approach used was innovative, based on competencies and skills, and because the teachers who would carry out the practice with the students were professionals working in hospitals and health units, that is, practically an education at work, as one of the teachers who worked with the indigenous people pointed out.

The idea of training indigenous people as nursing assistants and technicians did not come from the University, but from the cacique of the Xapecó Indigenous Land, Orides Belino C. da Silva. The cacique approached the UFSC requesting vacancies for indigenous people in the higher education course in nursing, but as it was impossible to meet this specific demand, the training of nursing technicians was proposed through the "Pioneer Project".

> This request was very interesting because, well, the cacique at the time, until later he was assassinated, it was a complicated thing there, and he had a perspective, a vision ahead of his time that was later consolidated in the system of affirmative action, because, what he came to ask for, at the time, in fact, were vacancies for the nursing course, vacancies for the higher education course. At the time, we were not aware of the possibility of having vacancies, neither for students from public schools, nor for blacks, nor for indigenous people, but he already wanted at that time, he made a demand for the

> university, as there was no such possibility, which at that time was only for university graduates, by vestibular, or transfer, which is also by vestibular. Anyway, Professor Claudete, who coordinated and still coordinates Repensul, made this counter-offer to create a special group for a technical nursing course for the indigenous people of their villages, of the Xapecó Indigenous Territory, for their approval as auxiliaries and technicians. He accepted and it was very important, because it was not an initiative of the university, it was a response to a specific demand from the indigenous people. It was very timely, like many things that Professor Claudete does, that historical, social and cultural reading. It was very important, because then this group was consolidated, which was only one group, one group of students in this modality (Professor Claudia of the UFSC).

According to the reports of the indigenous people who participated in the

"Pioneer Project" and information contained in their respective diplomas[15] , the course offered by the UFSC took place in two Modules. Module I - Nursing Assistant - had four units, totaling 1,110 hours, of which 400 hours were supervised internship (for a list of the disciplines, see Annex 4). Module II - Nursing Technician - offered two more units, with a total of 1,800 hours, of which 690 hours were supervised internship (for a list of subjects, see Annex 5). It should be noted that technical courses must present a minimum workload required for each area, which in the case of health is 1,200 hours.

The contents of Module I were basically related to biomedical care, but in Unit 2, which dealt with the contextualization of the nursing professional in the social environment, the subject "Regional Studies" was offered, when the "local customs and habits" of the indigenous people of the T.I. Xapecó were studied. For these classes, the oldest members of the T.I. were called in, as connoisseurs of medicinal plants, healers, folk healers, shamans, healers, as well as Sister Sara, involved in Pastoral Work, to teach about the medicinal plants and to report on the local "ancestral" medicine. These course guests would take the students into the bush to teach them how to recognise the plants, as well as how to collect and prepare them.

> During the auxiliary course we had a class on phytotherapies one day a week at the head office. Sister Sara guided us with the herbs. Dona Madalena and Catarina were called to help in the research of forest plants. And Mr José died this year at the age of 109, in the beginning of January [2011], he also used to do garrafada, benzimento and also helped with the course (Techn. Ind. Enf. Amanda).

In Module II, the study was directed to the hospital environment, with the aim of preparing these professionals to receive and offer specific attention to indigenous patients in this space, making it less strange and more familiar to those who leave their community to be attended to in the city. This was the intention of the hospital training for the indigenous technician:

> The good thing would be that professional who already has that load of good knowledge, who already knows the habits of each one, each one's approach, to work with. My concern is that a recently graduated technician cannot go to the hospital, because the teams will mould them in their own way. He needs to have about 4/5 years of knowledge of the people, to know the families" (Technician Ind. Enf Fernando).

The selection for the two modules did not include tests: the choices were made by affinity with the theme to be studied and by indication. There were two cases in which, due to the proximity with the cacique of the Indigenous Land, the choice was only by indication of the leadership.

Eight nursing assistants graduated, who went on to study nursing technical courses, with the addition of two more students. Among the ten graduates, four are hired as technicians; one had never worked as a technician, but had been working in health management in the T.I. Xapecó - at the time of the research he was unemployed; two others are unemployed due to political differences with the leadership; two are employed in

other functions (AIS and general services); and one is in Curitiba doing a higher education course.

3.2.4 Training and other courses held by nursing auxiliaries and technicians

When asked about the frequency of training and other courses, all technicians and assistants expressed liking to participate in such events, but complained that they are not very frequent: the last course held was on Oral Health, in November 2010 in the municipality of Ipuaçu. All the trainings they attended were free of charge. Table 4 lists the training courses held by three of these professionals, the only ones who provided all the diplomas and certificates of proof.

Through the interviews, it was observed that several had taken training courses on medicinal plants/ herbs/ herbal medicine. However, in the field research it was noted that only three of them have been putting their knowledge into practice and guiding the community in the use of herbs, as detailed below.

Practically all of the training courses offered by Funasa and by Ipuaçu and Entre Rios are attended by the professionals. The middle level professionals believe that it is important to take courses and keep up to date, according to Nursing Assistant Lucrécia: "I would like more training, so that I don't stand still.

Table 4 - Training carried out by three mid-level professionals, Xapecó Indigenous Land, SC.

Professional	Year	Course	Hourly load
Indigenous nursing technician Luana	1978	Nursing Attendant	80 hours (approx.)
	2002	Distance Learning Occupational Health and Safety	4 hours
	2005	Round table "Professional Ethics: a duty for all at the service of life".	2 hours (approx.)
	2007	Funasa: Training Workshop on Food and Nutrition Surveillance	32 hours

Nursing Auxiliary Lucrécia	1988	Nursing Auxiliary Technician (correspondence teaching)	Six months
	1993	State Conference on Health for Indigenous Peoples	12 hours
	1995	Communicable disease training;	36 hours
	1997	1st State Meeting on Health Education for Indigenous Peoples of SC	40 hours
	1998	1ª Training workshop for multipliers of the project: "Prevention of STDs and AIDS among the indigenous population of SC	24 hours
	1998	First Meeting on Public Health	24 hours
	1998	Basic Course in Phytotherapy	40 hours
	1998	Co-infection training course	24 hours
	1999	Introduction to Phytotherapy	24 hours
	2001	Medicinal Herbs	60 hours
	2002	Distance Learning Occupational Health and Safety	64 hours
	2002	II Regional Seminar on Safety and Health at Work	2 days
	2007	Second Training Course on Combating Drug Use and Alcoholism	20 days
	2008	Capacity Building on Alcoholism	8 hours
Nursing Technician Fernando	1999/ 2000	Indigenous Sanitation Agent Training Course	240 hours
	2004	Pastoral da Criança Leader's Guide	40 hours
	2005	Phytotherapy & Alternative Therapies Course	45 hours
	2005	Vaccine room training course	40 hours
	2006	Pedagogical Training for Facilitators of the Basic Professional Education Course for Indigenous Health Agents	42 hours
	2006	IV District Indigenous Health Conference	80 hours

	2006	Co-facilitators of the Pedagogical Training Course for Facilitators of Basic Professional Education for Indigenous Health Agents	40 hours
	2006	Co-Facilitator of the Basic Professional Education Course for Indigenous Health Agents - Intestinal Parasitosis and Skin Diseases Module	80 hours
	2006	Co-Facilitator of the Basic Professional Education Course for Indigenous Health Agents - Adult Health and Emergency Care Module	16 hours
	2007	Capacity Building Workshop on Food and Nutrition Surveillance	32 hours
	2007	Capacity Building for Local Indigenous Health Councillors	32 hours

3.3 Activities performed by nursing auxiliaries and technicians

The activities developed by technicians and assistants do not differ in practice. However, we must emphasize that the work process takes place at the primary care level, differently from secondary or tertiary care.

The Law for the Professional Exercise of Nursing, Law n° 7.498/86, article 23, establishes that (BRASIL, 1987):

> (...) the personnel who are performing nursing tasks, due to the lack of medium-level human resources in this area, without having specific training regulated by law, will be authorized by the Federal Council of Nursing to exercise elementary nursing activities (p. 06).

The sole paragraph of this article states: "The authorisation referred to in this article, which will follow the criteria established by the Federal Council of Nursing, can only be granted during the period of 10 (ten) years as of the promulgation of this Law", that is, until the year 1996. This paragraph was altered by Law n° 8.967/1994, mentioning that the nursing attendant admitted before this Law came into effect is assured the exercise of the elementary activities of these professionals.

The Ministry of Health sought to resolve this issue through Profae, which aimed to provide improvement in the quality of nursing care in health services. The project served to qualify the professionals already employed in health establishments through the complementation of basic education and professional qualification of the nursing assistant. As of 2002, the project incorporated the course on Complementation of the Professional Qualification of Nursing Assistant to Nursing Technician, due to the changes in the National Curricular Guidelines for Technical Level Professional Education for professionals who had already completed high school (COSTA et al., 2009).

Until shortly before the implementation of the subsystem in the T.I. Xapecó by FUNASA, health care was provided by nursing auxiliaries and assistants hired by FUNAI and by the mobile health teams (EVS), which made periodic visits to the villages for emergency care and immunisation, as seen in the chapter "Trajectory and methodology". Thus, the activities performed were different from those performed today, as stated by an indigenous person who has already worked as an attendant, as an auxiliary and today is hired as a nursing technician:

> At that time you had the nursing attendant to teach you how to do, sutures, deliveries, you did everything, not today, but back then it was. The attendant was the doctor, in that countryside. At that time, when a pregnant woman arrived, we did not take her to hospital, first because there was no hospital nearby, then because we had no car and the road was horrible. Today we have a good road, we have a car, we have a hospital, but at that time we did not have one, so we 'interned' at the clinic and assisted. We delivered babies, we medicated, we administered IVs, we took care of them (indigenous nurse technician Carlos).

At that time, the Federal Council of Nursing (Cofen) allowed attendants and auxiliaries to perform these activities when there were no duly authorised human resources in the distant and/or indigenous villages, as mentioned above.

However, as today there are professionals formed and trained to perform specific activities, according to Decree n° 94.406/86 which regulates Law n° 7.498/86, and as the organization of services is regulated (BRASIL, 1987 and 2007), there remains the memory of those older ones, when they were allowed to act in the most diverse activities:

> So, we have been working this way, but since that law, of the nursing council, which has that discussion from 1988, that says that an auxiliary is an auxiliary, a technician is a technician and a nurse is a nurse, that prevents us from doing the procedures that we used to do, doing more things, the procedures that we used to do. I had more responsibility, today there is the nurse who has this responsibility (Technician Ind. Nurse Carlos).

The activities of assistants, according to Cofen, are actions of a basic level and repetitive nature, "involving auxiliary Nursing services under supervision, as well as participation at the level of simple execution, in treatment processes, with special responsibility for: observing, recognising and describing signs and symptoms; performing simple treatment actions; providing hygiene care and comfort to the patient; participating in the health team" as provided for in Article 13 of Law n° 7.498/86 (BRASIL, 1986, pp. 4-5).

In a hospital setting, this would translate exactly into the actions described above, which are simple and basic activities, such as hygiene, comfort and observation of signs and symptoms. However, in primary care, the actions differ from those in the hospital environment, and the auxiliary gains more responsibilities in the health posts. Their attributions are accompany the nursing consultations when requested, especially in the consultations to individuals exposed to situations of risk, aiming to ensure a better monitoring of their health conditions; perform together with the community health agents the identification of families at risk and contribute, when requested, with their work in home visits; execute, according to their professional qualification, the procedures of sanitary and epidemiological surveillance in the areas of care to children, women, adolescents, workers, and the elderly, as well as in the control of tuberculosis, leprosy, chronic degenerative and infectious diseases; and participate in the discussion and organization of the work process of the health unit (BRAZIL, 1997, p. 17). 17).

The activities of nursing technicians, according to article 12 of Law no.° 7.498/86, involve the orientation and supervision of nursing work "to an auxiliary degree, and participation in the planning of nursing care, with special responsibility for: participating in the programming of nursing care; executing nursing care actions, except those exclusive to nurses, in accordance with the provisions of the sole paragraph of article 11 of this Law; participating in the orientation and supervision of nursing work to an auxiliary degree and participating in the health team" (BRASIL, 1986, pp. 4-5).

The nursing technician should perform functions of greater responsibility than the 'auxiliary, such as lecturing, caring for the vaccine room and planning nursing actions together with the nurse, and may also perform the Papanicolau examination (preventive of cervical cancer) in the Women's Health Program, provided that they are trained and accompanied by direct supervision by the nurse (BRASIL, 1986).

Despite the fact that the actions of the technician and the assistant are defined according to the legislation, it was observed that in the practice of the I.T. Xapecó, the activities of the mid-level indigenous professionals exceed the attributions described above. Among the activities carried out by mid-level professionals at the posts of the I.T. Xapecó it was observed:

- carrying out dressings;

- cleaning and organising nursing equipment;
- sterilisation of dressing material;
- checking temperature, blood pressure, weight and height;
- delivery of prescription drugs;
- delivery of medicines without medical prescription, meeting user demand;
- administration of prescribed oral medicines;
- administration of non-prescribed oral medication on demand;
- administration of injectable drugs with a doctor's prescription;
- administration of injectable drugs without medical prescription, meeting user demand;
- indication and administration of medication;
- administration of serotherapy;
- assistance in urgencies and emergencies;
- assistance in guiding ISAs;
- providing inhalation and nebulisation to the patient;
- organisation of nursing supplies;
- organisation and control of medicine stock;
- help in scheduling exams and specialised consultations;
- carrying out visits;
- assistance to bedridden patients in their homes;
  guidance and administration of remedies based on medicinal plants (teas, shampoos, ointments, soaps, syrups, etc.).

It draws attention, again, that there is no difference in the activities carried out by technicians or assistants, except when it comes to medicinal plants. In the posts where there are nurses, the coordination and local administration of activities is delegated to these professionals, thus restricting the activities of technicians and assistants to technical and guidance functions.

There is one health post, distant from the one in the main village, which has an indigenous nursing technician and an AIS. In this post, the nursing technician coordinates the local activities, including: the organization of the agenda of medical appointments that take place once a week during the morning period; organization of home visits; provision of general services to the community; organization, cleaning and storage of inputs and medicines.

In another post, where no doctor was hired and working during the research period and where there is an indication for the use of plants from the medicinal garden, the nursing technician provides assistance to the community: sometimes with medicines, sometimes with herbal remedies prepared in the post itself. The indigenous technician of this post also works in the Health Pastoral and the Children's Pastoral and has the help of the Catholic Church and the sisters of a religious congregation. Even with this help, she coordinates all the actions related to the medicinal garden and the manufacturing of medicines with the help of community volunteers and some AIS from the health post. This nursing technician instructs the AIS to take care of the garden and produce herbal remedies, as well as giving Pastoral Health leadership training courses to the community. It should be noted that the activity involving medicinal plants was only carried out systematically in this post during the research period, although there are medicinal gardens in at least two other villages in the Indigenous Land, which were not receiving maintenance. The revitalization of the gardens is well regarded by doctors, nurses and dentists, who think it is "great that the culture is being rescued".

It should be noted that most indigenous nursing auxiliaries and technicians have training courses on medicinal plants, mostly sponsored by the Pastoral Health Care, including care and cultivation, among other topics related to the theme, as discussed below. Langdon and Diehl (2007) point out that the Pastoral encouraged the use of medicinal herbs by the Kaingáng, which had been gaining strength in recent decades. Even so, after some time, the use of herbs and the care of the medicinal garden were practices left in the background in most health posts:

> In 2004, the Health Post of the Aldeia Sede had a medicinal garden and a small laboratory for processing medicinal plants, under the command of a technical attendant with several years of experience. In addition to being considered a "specialist" by the Kaingang people and serving patients at the Health Post, this EMSI employee also trained other indigenous people in the processing of teas, ointments and infusions. This knowledge was replicated throughout the community by means of the AISs and volunteer health agents of the Pastoral. Coupled with the use of these products, there was a whole ideological construction by society in which they were instruments for "rescuing traditional indigenous medical culture". Unfortunately, in 2006 we found the 'bush pharmacy' practically abandoned, the laboratory unavailable and the specialist in the process of returning to her original function as a dentist's assistant at the village Health Post" (pp. 26-27).

It was observed that both the patient/user seeks the nursing technician/assistant when arriving at the station, and also before leaving, as the professional receives him/her, going to his/her aid and, according to the demands, performing the first procedures, such as triage, defining what should be done, and/or the pre-consultation, when temperature, blood pressure, weight and height are measured. After the consultation, the patient receives, mainly from the technician/auxiliary, the medication and/or care prescribed by the physician (dressings, administration of medication, inhalation, etc.).

Even when there is no doctor in the unit, the technician or assistant receives the patient and assists him/her in his/her demands (delivery of material, medication, administration of intramuscular contraceptive, etc.). When there is a need for a more significant intervention, for example, in the case of a very high fever, or a convulsion, or very high blood pressure, this professional calls the nurse, who will provide the necessary support.

To illustrate this situation, we quote a case observed in the field: a mother arrives at the clinic with a child on her lap, and the nursing assistant asks what happened. The mother reports that the child has a high fever. The indigenous auxiliary asks her to sit with the child in her lap while she puts the thermometer on; when she verifies that the temperature is over 39°C, the professional calls the nurse, who, after asking the mother more questions, asks the indigenous auxiliary to apply cold compresses and administer dipyrone drops according to the child's weight, leaving the child under observation. After a while, as the fever did not give way, the nurse called a car to take the child to the reference hospital in Xanxerê, a municipality close to the Indigenous Land.

However, when neither the nurse nor the doctor are present, and depending on the gravity of the situation and the time of the occurrence, the professionals at the post take the patient with the FUNASA car to another village post that has a doctor or to the reference hospital.

The mid-level professionals must also work with the team in the actions of the Women's Health, Child Health, Adolescent Health, Adult Health, Worker's Health, Elderly Health, Oral Health, Nutritional Health, Mental Health, Emergencies, Epidemiological Surveillance, Vaccination, Chronic Degenerative Diseases and Communicable Diseases programs. Among the activities that must be performed by these professionals in these programs are: with the help of the AIS, identify the families/people who must participate in the orientation meetings organized; assist in weighing and measuring vital data of patients/community; assist the team in urgencies and emergencies; assist/perform lectures together with the AIS in the community; conduct visits, among others.

It is reaffirmed that, in practice, auxiliaries and technicians act in a similar way in all contexts, that is, this is not a practice that occurs within indigenous lands, but throughout Brazil. Peduzzi and Anselmi (2004) emphasize, in the report on the impact of the Profae:

> In the three services studied, the description of the activities of nursing auxiliaries and technicians allows us to observe that it is the same work, there is no distinction in the actions or interventions that both professionals perform. All the interviewed nursing auxiliaries and technicians clearly and objectively stated that they do not identify any effective

difference in the work they carry out, that is, there are no differences in the daily exercise of the work of both categories. In most of the statements given by physicians, there is also no difference between the work performed by nursing auxiliaries or nursing technicians (') In the nurses' reports, there are also no differences between the work performed by nursing auxiliaries and nursing technicians. One of the maternity nurses mentions that "assistants with many years of experience are better than technicians who are graduating" and that, in the study unit, there are no criteria or parameters to distinguish both jobs. Thus, it is observed that, in addition to the lack of objective differences between the work performed by auxiliaries and technicians, for both professionals there is an expressive valuation of practical work experience as a criterion for professional performance (p. 70).

When interviewed, nursing assistants and technicians stated that, in practice, all perform the same activities. If, eventually, there is a division of work, it happens by affinity, not by professional category.

There are technicians involved with other activities not described as being within the competence of their profession. As already mentioned, there is one technician who works with the Pastoral and two others who are very active in social control. Both have already been presidents of the Local Indigenous Health Council and another is still a member of the Southern Interior Indigenous Health District Council. The view of one of them on the work of indigenous professionals is described below:

> Who does good work is the professional, who makes things happen depends on us, on each one of us, but it doesn't matter, for example, I don't get angry if they tell me to work in another way to see if things change. And I have to do it, we have to be open to change, to become better. Because I came to the conclusion today that things are going too fast, but it is not because things are going too fast that they are being run over that we have to take it this way. We have to stop and evaluate. Here in our post office there are many difficulties, I have to take care of the post office, the medication; do the role of a janitor, clean the post every Friday; I have to take care of the file, visit the post office. I control the hypertensive patients (Tec. Ind. Enf. Fernando).

This technician is a professional who, generally, when there are conflicts that require the intervention of leaders or major decisions, is requested to participate in mediations.

According to the community, to become a good health professional, one has to be very patient in dealing with Indians, as one service user points out: "You have to be gentle. He has to be humble and have patience with the little Indian who comes to the clinic and sits quietly in the corner. You have to know how to talk and get through to them" (Maria).

When comparing the activities of the indigenous nursing technician and those of the AIS, one can see that they are very different. The AIS basically carries out home visits and fills out countless forms. According to Langdon and Diehl (2007), "the home visits and their registration on forms made the activities ambiguous and without clear justification for the agents. Faced with prohibitions to perform primary care, they expressed the confrontation of contradictory expectations from EMSI and the community" (p. 24).

According to a technician who has served as an ISA for four years:

> AIS has to be close to the community and a technician is more about disease prevention/lectures and serving people in the clinic. I like both professions, but the wage difference made me choose to be a technician. I like the actions of the nursing technician, such as dressings, IM - IV - SC applications, checking blood pressure. The coolest part of the profession is the pleasure of working with the people, see them open up and help, in the beginning there is fear, fear and then trust. It's great and the worst part is that there are many people for specialized consultations and this takes time, and not being able to help is very bad and the suffering of waiting is bad. The people are needy. (Indigenous Nursing Technician Gabriel)

3.4 Turnover of health professionals at T.I. Xapecó

This is a problem that is not restricted to indigenous populations; the turnover of indigenous and non-indigenous professionals occurs throughout the country. Just as there is turnover in the T. I. Xapecó, there is turnover in several other Special Indigenous Health Districts, according to Garnelo et al. (2003), Langdon and Diehl (2007), Novo (2010), among others. This interruption of work brings dissatisfaction not only for the team, but for the community as it makes it impossible or breaks a possible bond.

This turnover is related to many factors, among them: the non-adaptation of non-indigenous professionals to working with indigenous populations, the lack of adequate training to work in inter-ethnic contexts, among others. As well as the "cultural" issue and its understanding is perhaps the main difficulty faced by health professionals in providing care to indigenous peoples. According to Langdon and Diehl (2007):

> The notions of culture and traditional medicine tend to be conceptualised in the 'museum' mould, seeking cultural traits, homogeneity and integrity that do not exist. Professionals fail

> to recognise that the boundaries between official health services and the practices of indigenous medicines are permeable (p. 31).

As far as indigenous professionals are concerned, one of the reasons is linked to internal and external political processes, according to Langdon and Diehl (2007):

> Between May and July 2004, for example, we found that practically 50% of the teams at T. I. Xapecó had been changed. Both the AISs and the other members of the EMSIs were constantly being replaced, either for political reasons or for not adapting to the rhythm, dynamics and pressures that mark the daily exercise of their functions. The causes of the high turnover of AISs were related in part to the ways in which AISs were hired and selected, both of which were marked by political processes internal and external to I.T. (p. 23).

More recently (between August 2010 and February 2011), it was possible to observe that AIS were dismissed and rehired without there being a change. The indigenous health agents had been dismissed for a new hiring via a selection process in January 2011. In the selection notice, one of the requirements pointed out the need for certification of the refresher course for ISAs, held by the Entre Rios City Hall in agreement with the Health Training School (EFOS) the previous year (training in 2010), limiting entry to professionals who already worked in this function, which facilitated the work of the teams: "It is a difficulty to change health agents, we have to start all over again, we train, train and then change everything again, and then change when the cacique changes" (Techn. Ind. Enf. Amanda).

During the fieldwork period, the professionals' contract with the partner[16] had already expired and was being extended for the second time at the time of my leaving the area.

The insecurity about the rehiring, which included the fear that it might not occur, was a constant conversation in the professionals' meetings during the working day. Another reason for insecurity was based on the transition of indigenous health management from Funasa to Sesai, as previously commented. "I wanted it to improve in general, that I could present: this is my work here. I wanted the working conditions to improve" (General service assistant Luana).

The professional says she wanted stability so she could show her work with security. This line demonstrates the anguish experienced at each termination and renewal of contract and how much it upsets them because there is no stability, reducing the chances of them taking other training courses.

In the case of indigenous nursing technicians and auxiliaries, it is observed that there is no significant turnover, and some of them have worked in health for many years, although dissatisfaction with the constant terminations and rehiring is present.

3.5 The role of nursing auxiliaries and technicians at T.I. Xapecó

In the EMSI, the nursing technician/assistant, after the AIS, is the professional who has the greatest contact with the population. Their activities are more complex than those delegated to the agents and, in some cases, they assume the local coordination of the health post, as is the case in one of the villages of the T.I. Xapecó. Despite taking on more complex tasks than the ISA, the technician carries out fewer bureaucratic activities than the agent.

The activities performed by the indigenous professional are the same as those required of non-indigenous professionals of the same category. In addition, they also assume the role of facilitator, translator, interlocutor between the health team and the community. This function is clearly visible to those who observe them working in the health posts in the villages.

The team perceives them as the interlocutor of medical and curative recommendations, as well as of the anxieties and fears of patients who do not want to undergo some medical procedure. The indigenous technician and auxiliary intervenes in order to make the patient and/or his caregiver accept and comply with the biomedical recommendation. Sometimes, however, the user expresses his own understanding of the situation, as shown in the following account:

A lady comes to the clinic complaining of a "ball" in her belly. She presents with a large bulge in her abdomen that looks like a folded garment under the blouse she is wearing. The nurse asks the indigenous auxiliary nurse to lay her down on a stretcher in the observation room. The auxiliary nurse returns saying that the "ball" disappears when the woman lies down. The nurse goes to the room, and the doctor arrives next. As she lifted up her blouse, the doctor palpated her, checking for a scar; he asked her if she had ever had surgery on her stomach, to which she nodded. He then makes the diagnosis and, looking at the attendant, says: "After an abdominal surgery, the necessary care was not taken, the stitches broke and she has a large abdominal hernia". The doctor looks at the lady lying down and says: "Now there is only one thing to do". The lady completes, "Yes, now there is only one thing to do, the hip sympathy has to do". The doctor smiles and adds: "Now there is only another surgery with the placement of a mesh in the abdomen". So, the lady went home and the nurse scheduled exams for a new surgery.

In the doctor's words, it is noted that the community's care practices are not considered, which shows how unprepared they are
non-indigenous professionals facing a new reality, as Diehl (2001a) states in his work:

In another situation, the nursing technician was performing a dressing on
a boy who had had a motorbike accident over the weekend. During the dressing,
Gabriel jokingly said: "What happened, home? Did you have *a few drinks* and
fall off the bike? The boy, smiling, confirms with his head that yes. Noting that
the stitches (on the left lumbar, at the level of the kidney) were becoming
infected, Gabriel told the boy to get medicine at the pharmacy, asking if he had
a prescription. The boy again confirms that he does, and the technician asks him
to take it in order not to infect the wound: "But you have to stop *drinking* while
you are taking the medicine," he concludes with a smile, and the boy returns the
smile, saying nothing.

In this other situation, the indigenous professional noticed the cause of the
injuries (drunkenness that caused the accident) and, by indicating the treatment
asking him to "stop drinking", shows us the subtlety with which the indigenous
professional guides the patient to stay without drinking during the period in
which he is taking medication.

These situations show us that, despite the medical indications, the
community also has its own way of dealing with the situations experienced, as
NOVO (2010) states in his work:

Ferraz (2010), studying among the Kaingáng people of western Santa
Catarina, noticed that the concepts of health and illness of health professionals
are based on biomedicine knowledge, while the indigenous people base their
health care on popular knowledge. The professionals, concerned with hygiene
issues learned from the biomedicine perspective, worry about the fact that the
indigenous people do not share the same perceptions, and for this reason the
families' care "compromises" the health of their children.

> own beliefs, values and relationships with nature. The concern
> of professionals with the hygiene of indigenous children is
> related to their vulnerability to falling ill, according to the
> bases of biomedicine (FERRAZ, 2010, p. 83).

For Ferraz (2010), the presence of indigenous people as nursing technicians is a possibility to change this situation: "However, the presence of three indigenous nursing technicians shows that there is already a sensitivity to the need for a culturally congruent care" (FERRAZ, 2010, p. 85).

In this way, it is possible to observe the search for professional training of the indigenous people who, through professionalization, learn to care for the community and try to find a balance between technical and popular care.

It is a fact that professionals need time to get to know and understand the local care practices (with time not being, for some professionals, the only factor necessary for this understanding/comprehension). However, the turnover of professionals is high, as discussed above, and thus the non-indigenous members of the EMSI do not create a link or maintain contact with the diversity of existing knowledge, so that they could learn to respect and articulate it.

> It is important to highlight here the great difficulty for
> professionals to find the balance between the duties of their
> professional culture and the respect for the other's culture.
> When informants describe care, it is clear that the professional
> duty ends up prevailing, and thus the cultural imposition of
> care occurs (FERRAZ, 2010, pp. 97-98).

The indigenous professional values the role of interlocutor, as he sees himself as the "caretaker" of the community, perceiving the importance of his explanations or of his intervention with the community. In addition, it facilitates access to some resources, such as medicines, which can be dispensed without the presentation of a prescription, as shown in the following situation.

A lady arrives at the clinic on an afternoon when the doctors are not present. All the indigenous technicians and assistants and a non-indigenous nurse are working. The lady enters and looks for the indigenous nursing technician: "I have a lot of pain in my arm, Gabriel. Can you give me an injection? Diclofenac? "Lady: "That's fine."

This description illustrates how the community, in turn, sees the indigenous nursing worker as someone accessible, helpful, ready to exercise care; he is a familiar person with the rest of the health team, whom they can ask for an explanation on how and when to take medication or receive support when hospital removal is necessary.

Non-Indigenous professionals also point out this difference: that Indigenous professionals tend to be much calmer and more thoughtful than non-

Indigenous professionals:

> Working in a white area is worse than in the reserve, in the white area there is always someone who says 'I know more than you, you know nothing'. (...) It is much nicer to work in the reserve, the population, the people know how to respect us much more than the white population. And in the team there is more, they are more human (non-indigenous nursing technician Leda).

The indigenous health professional is well seen by the team. EMSI perceives the community professionals as "allies" in the argumentation with the community and recognizes that their relationship with the community is much better. Thus, the training of indigenous health professionals is quite important, and the team recognizes the qualities of empathy and serenity in the care provided by these professionals.

> Indigenous nursing technicians are more reserved than non-Indigenous technicians (...) I am not an Indian, they are more open with the population, and in this openness I insert myself (...) the people have respect, because they live in the community (...) they trust a lot, sometimes they come and ask for Anastacia, or for Chico, because they feel more comfortable (...) the community feels more comfortable with the indigenous technicians, even among themselves (Nurse Laura).

> Indigenous technicians are well dedicated (...) have more patience, are more sincere, calmer, the non-indigenous nursing technicians, what they do with more perfection, more technique, but the indigenous are more intelligent (Nurse Laura).

Some mention that they learned to slow down the previously frenetic pace of care with the indigenous professionals, who are generally considered very calm: "With the indigenous technician there is no difficulty, on the contrary, he is calmer, he is not worried about hierarchy at work (...) they are very calm, they even taught me how to calm down" (Nurse Laila).

In the daily work process, the supervision of indigenous professionals is slightly more accentuated than that of non-indigenous professionals. This is due to the constant requests for help from the indigenous technicians/assistants to the nurses or the doctor. It also occurs because they believe that the indigenous people's schooling "was weak", so there is insecurity in invasive procedures.

> They are not very secure, they are a little more dependent. I think because they had a 'weaker' school since they were

children, that makes it a little difficult, but even so... (...) all the activities are together, I go with them wherever they need me. They do everything, sometimes they have difficulty doing something, but then we help them, and they do it very well after we show them (Nurse Laura).

On the other hand, an indigenous nursing technician, who has completed higher education but works as a technician, has an important view on the training of indigenous people in health:

There is a lack of trained indigenous professionals. There is a faculty to train indigenous people, but only in the area of education, and not in the area of health. This college is a partnership between UNIOESTE and UFSC, with classes every 15 days one weekend in Chapecó. Friday night and Saturday all day. There are buses that take and bring, there are some that are doing it. But it needs in the area of health (Anastacia, indigenous nursing technician).

(...) the plants have their healing effect, but now that the Indians eat industrialized products, not only bush/natural food anymore, they need to be cured with medicines from the pharmacy, besides the teas, because their diet has changed and now only bush medicines do not help alone, they also need hypertension and diabetes medicine (...) those who are in the health post and do not have this knowledge of the indigenous community suffer because they do not know (Anastacia, indigenous nursing technician).

This technician also points out that when professionals give lectures, they do not know how to put the examples into local reality, and thus do not "convince" everyone to follow their guidance on disease prevention:

Team does not understand the local leaders, customs and healers (...) the hypertension lectures in the community, for example, they talk about the technical issue and then invite Ms. Madalena to talk about medicinal plants and teas that help to improve. Madalena's talks made them understand that they were hypertensive because of their diet, which used to be all natural and now there are a lot of industrialized products that don't help the teas to have their effect, and there is also the issue that the plants are very agrotoxic, which is why it is necessary to include medication in the treatment of hypertension. It is necessary to convince the indigenous people. Lectures only with non-indigenous professionals are not convincing because they do not have the community's understanding (Anastacia, indigenous nursing technician).

CHAPTER 4

Final considerations

The Kaingáng are a people who live in the west of Santa Catarina, but are still located from the southwest of São Paulo to the northwest of Rio Grande do Sul, inhabiting a region of intense contact with non-Indians, where "they establish interethnic relations that are so complex that it is difficult to find discrete cultural patterns" (DIEHL, 2001a, p. 162).

The "cultural" issue and its understanding is perhaps the main difficulty faced by health professionals in caring for indigenous peoples. Thus, there is a need for approximation between public health and anthropology, which has been increasing in recent decades. However, there is still a mistaken view of culture, which is systematically used by professionals and managers to justify a "non-compliance" by the groups assisted with biomedical recommendations.

In the West, the biomedical model has assumed a dominant position over other medical systems not only because of its efficacy, but also as a result of the expansion of the capitalist economy throughout the world. However, the interaction between biomedicine and indigenous medicines generates a process of reconstruction of knowledge and practices. The boundaries between different medical knowledge are fluid and generate a space of intermedicality (FÓLLER, 2004), which is not a homogeneous space, but rather a variable, continuous and dynamic process.

Leininger (1991) develops a theory that unites anthropology and nursing, through the respect for "cultural diversities", and adds that in this globalised world, where transformations and contacts with people from different realities occur all the time, it is necessary that nursing is attentive to better understand and assist individuals in their most vulnerable moments, respecting the differences of understanding about health, disease, care, well-being and death. Nursing must study and understand the different ways of perceiving these factors in order to better assist people, besides understanding that without understanding, there will be no comprehension on both sides of the care to be provided, which can cause great frustration, confusion and anger. At this moment, theory gains relevance in helping to understand the differences.

The insertion of the indigenous health agent was intended to mediate between the health services and indigenous knowledge, as well as between the members of the health team and the communities
attended to. The "differentiated attention" in the model of indigenous health care implemented in 1999 by the Ministry of Health gives more prominence to the AIS. Recent studies, such as those already cited, point to the dissatisfaction of the AIS and stimulate the search for professional courses for nursing assistants and technicians for a greater insertion in the EMSI, or for salary issues, or even

for definitions of the activities to be exercised.

In the EMSI, the nursing technician/assistant, after the AIS, is the professional who has the greatest contact with the population. He/she performs more complex activities than the agent and, in some cases, assumes the local coordination of the health post, as is the case in one of the villages of the T.I. Xapecó. Despite taking on more complex tasks than the AIS, they perform fewer bureaucratic functions than the agent. The activities carried out by the indigenous professional are the same as those required of a non-indigenous professional of the same category. In addition, they also assume the role of facilitator/translator/interlocutor between the health team and the community. This function is clearly visible to those who observe them working in the health post. The team perceives him as the interlocutor of medical/curative recommendations, as well as of the anxieties and fears of patients who do not want to undergo some medical procedure.

The indigenous technician/auxiliary intervenes in order to make the patient and/or his/her caregiver accept and comply with the biomedical recommendation. The indigenous professional values this role of interlocutor, as he sees himself as the "caretaker" of the community, perceiving the importance of his explanations or of his intervention with the community. The community, in turn, sees him as someone accessible, helpful, ready to provide care; he is a relative together with the rest of the health team, to whom they can ask for an explanation about how and when to take medication, make a compress, or even give support when it is necessary to go to hospital. In addition, it facilitates access to some resources, such as medicines, which can be dispensed without the presentation of a prescription.

In the T.I. Xapecó there were 16 indigenous people with a medium level degree in nursing, ten of whom were effectively working in a function compatible with their training, carrying out activities linked to biomedical practice. However, there are few who carry out practices linked to the use of medicinal plants, despite all having received training in this area; there are few who show confidence in administering "bush remedies". However, EMSI professionals stress the importance of using local healing practices.

In relation to the vocational courses in which indigenous people participated, it can be observed that the biomedical model is impregnated in the curricula. Thus, there is no (or little) space for local knowledge and practices, i.e., they are still very far from including indigenous specificities.

In the perspective of continuing their training, there is a desire on the part of the technicians and assistants for a university education, especially in medicine (in second and third place come nursing and psychology respectively), which, according to them, would be to be able to integrate the curative practices of their community. Few feel willing to leave the village and go to other cities to pursue these courses. However, they affirm that if it were offered in a closer place they would take a higher education course. For the community, there is also an expectation that indigenous people study, seeking more specialized training, according to Maria and Catarina, community members, who express well the role of the indigenous nursing technician/auxiliary:

> You have to be gentle when dealing with Indians. You have to have patience, gentleness and a lot of love (...) He [referring to a nursing technician] was too intelligent to work in the sun [compared to the time when this Indian worked as a HIA]. It's good that he studied and he has to study more.

There is a long way to go regarding indigenous health and professional qualification courses aimed at training indigenous people. Considering the ethnic/cultural diversity of the country, it is necessary to have more studies and research directed to professional qualification issues considering the various existing ethnic groups.

This work does not intend to define how training courses should be carried out or structured. Intercultural dialogue may occur in a negotiated manner. This dialogue between the different interlocutors legitimizes and makes room for the knowledge of local communities during the process of building the professional qualification, respecting diversities. Thus, it will be possible to change the process of construction of curricula of health courses aimed at indigenous populations.

REFERENCE

ALMEIDA, L. **Análise antropológica das igrejas cristãs entre os Kaingang baseada na etnografia, na cosmologia e dualismo**. Thesis (Doctorate in Social Anthropology), Federal University of Santa Catarina, Florianópolis, 2004.

BALDUS, H. **Ensaios de etnologia brasileira**. São Paulo: Cia. Ed. Nacional, 1937.

BOEHS, A. E. Análise dos conceitos de negociação/acomodação da teoria de M. Leininger. **Revista Latino-Americana de Enfermagem**, v. 10, n. 1, pp. 90-96,2002. Available at: <http://www.scielo.br/scielo.php?script=sci_arttext&pid=S0104-11692002000100014&lng=en&nrm=iso>. Accessed on: 10 Jun. 2011.

BRAZIL. Ministry of Health. Fundação Nacional de Saúde. **Política nacional de atenção à saúde dos povos indígenas**. 2. ed. Brasília: Fundação Nacional de Saúde, 2002a.

BRAZIL. **Law nº 10.507**, of July 10, 2002. Cria a profissão de Agente Comunitário de Saúde e dá outras providências. 2002b.
Available at:
<http://www6.senado.gov.br/legislacao/ListaPublicacoes.action?id=235 057>.
Accessed on: 3 May 2011.

BRAZIL. **Decree nº 94.406/1987**. Regulamenta a Lei nº 7.498/1986, que dispõe sobre o exercício profissional da Enfermagem. 1987.
Available at: <http://www.portalcofen.gov.br/sitenovo/node/4173>.
Accessed on: 3 May 2002.

BRASIL. National Indian Foundation. **Maps of Indigenous Lands in Santa Catarina**. 2011a . Available at: <http://mapas.funai.gov.br/>. Accessed on 05 May 2011.

BRAZIL. National Indian Foundation (Funai). **History of indigenous health**. 2011b. Available at:
<http://www.funai.gov.br/quem/historia/spi.htm>. Accessed on: 25 May 2011.

BRAZIL. **Decree No.º 7.530/2011**, revoking Decree No. 7.530/2011, on the transition of the management of the Indigenous Health Care Subsystem from the National Health Foundation to the Ministry of Health. 2011c. Available at:
<http://www.planalto.gov.br/ccivil_03/_Ato2011-2014/2011/Decreto/D7461.htm>. Accessed on: 3 May 2011.

BRAZIL. Ministry of Health. **Escolas Técnicas de Saúde**. 2011d.
Available at: <http://www.retsus.epsjv.fiocruz.br/index.php?Area=RETSUS>.
Accessed on: 5 May 2011.

BRAZIL. Ministry of Health. Fundação Nacional de Saúde. **Indigenous Health - Transition.** 2011. Available at:
<http://www.funasa.gov.br/internet/transicao/saudeIndigenaTransicao.as p>.
Accessed on: 3 May 2011.

BRAZIL. Ministry of Health. National Health Foundation.
RedeFunasa: **Number of people.** Data referring to July 1º , 2010. Available at:
<http://sis. funasa. gov.br/transparencia_publica/ siasiweb/Layout/quantita tivo_de_pessoas_2010.asp#>. Accessed on: 15 Mar. 2011.

BRASIL. Ministry of Health. **Projeto de Profissionalização dos Trabalhadores da área de Enfermagem (Profae)**, 2003a. Available at:
<http:// portal.saude. gov.br/portal/saude/profissional/visualizar_texto.cf m?idtxt=26827>. Accessed on: 4 May 2011.

BRASIL. Ministry of Health. **HumanizaSUS**. Política nacional de humanização do SUS. 2003b. Available at: <http://portal.saude. gov.br/portal/saude/cidadao/area.cfm?id_area=1342>. Accessed on: 2 jun. 2011.

BRAZIL. Ministry of Health. **The Project for the Professionalization of Workers in the Nursing Area**. Available at: <http://www.brasilsus.com.br/legislacoes/gm/734-1262>. Accessed on: 10 May 2011.

BRAZIL. Ministry of Health. **Ordinance No.º 2.656/2007**. Dispõe sobre as responsabilidades na prestação da atenção à saúde dos povos indígenas no Ministério da Saúde e regulamentação dos Incentivos de Atenção

Basic and Specialized to Indigenous Peoples. Diário Oficial da União, 18 oct. 2007.

BRAZIL. Ministry of Health. **Projeto de Profissionalização dos Trabalhadores da Área de Enfermagem**, Brasília, v. 2, n. 5, 2002.

BRAZIL. Ministry of Health. Secretariat of Health Assistance. Coordenação de Saúde da Comunidade. **Saúde da Família**: uma estratégia para a reorientação do modelo assistencial. Brasília, DF: Ministry of Health, 1997. Available at: <http://bvsms.saude.gov.br/bvs/publicacoes/cd09_16.pdf>. Accessed on 10 May2011.

BRAZIL. Ministry of Health. Secretariat of Health Surveillance. Programa Nacional de DST/AIDS. **Distritos Sanitários Especiais Indígenas**: Diretrizes para Implantar o Programa de DST/AIDS/ Ministério da Saúde, Secretaria de Vigilância em Saúde, Programa Nacional de DST/AIDS. Brasília: Ministry of Health, 2005.

CASTRO, C. M. G. L. **Projeto Xamã: o processo de formação e atuação dos auxiliares de enfermagem indígena Kurâ-Bakairi**. Dissertation (Master's in Collective Health), Federal University of Mato Grosso, Cuiabá, 2007.

CASTRO, T. G. de et al. Nutritional status of Kaingáng indigenous people enrolled in indigenous schools in the State of Rio Grande do Sul, Brazil. **Cadernos de Saúde Pública**, Rio de Janeiro, v. 26, n. 9, Sep. 2010. Available at: <http://www. scielosp. org/scielo. php?script=sci_arttext&pid=S0102-311X2010000900010&lng=en&nrm=iso>. Accessed on: 7 Oct. 2010.

COSTA, G. D.; COTTA, R. M. M.; FERREIRA, M. L. S. M.; REIS, J. R.;

FRANCESCHINI, S. C. C. Family health: challenges in the process of reorientation of the care model. **Revista Brasileira de Enfermagem**, Brasília, v. 62, n. 1, pp. 113-118, jan./feb. 2009.

CRÉPEAU, R. Mythe et rituel chez les indiens Kaingang du Brésil Méridional. **Religiologiques**, v. 10, pp. 143-157, 1994.

CROSSETTI, M. G. O.; SCOLA, M. L.; BUÓGO, M. O significado de cuidar na perspectiva de alunos de um Curso de Auxiliar de

Enfermagem. **Revista Gaúcha de Enfermagem**, Porto Alegre, v. 21, n. esp., pp. 56-69, 2000.

D'ANGELIS, V. R. Para uma História dos indios do Oeste Catarinense. In: **Cadernos do Centro de Organização da Memória Sócio-Cultural do Oeste de SC (CEOM)**. Chapecó, Santa Catarina, 1989.

DIAS-SCOPEL, R.; LANGDON, E.E.; SCOPEL, D. Emerging expectations: the insertion of the Xokleng indigenous health agent in the multidisciplinary indigenous health care team. **Tellus Journal**, v.[13,] pp. 51-73, 2008.

DIEHL, E. E. Agravos na saúde Kaingáng (Terra Indígena Xapecó, Santa Catarina State) e a estrutura dos serviços de atenção biomédica. **Cadernos de Saúde Pública**, Rio de Janeiro, v. 17, n.
2, Mar. 2001a. Available at:
<http:// www. scielosp. org/scielo. php? script=sci_arttext&pid=S0102-311X2001000200019&lng=en&nrm=iso>. Accessed on: 7 Oct. 2010.

DIEHL, E. E. **Entendimentos, práticas e contextos sociopolíticos de uso de medicamentos entre os Kaingáng (Terra Indígena Xapecó, Santa Catarina, Brasil)**. 2001. 246 f. Thesis (Doctorate in Public Health) - National School of Public Health, Oswaldo Cruz Foundation, Rio de Janeiro, 2001b.

FASSHEBER, J.R. **Saúde e Políticas de Saúde entre os Kaingáng de Palmas/PR**. 1998. 183 f. Dissertation (Master's in Anthropology) - Graduate Program in Social Anthropology, Universidade Federal de Santa Catarina, Florianópolis, 1998.

FERNANDES, R. C. **Autoridade política Kaingang: um estudo sobre a construção da legitimidade política entre os Kaingang de Palmas/Paraná.** Dissertation (Master's in Anthropology) - Graduate Program in Social Anthropology, Federal University of Santa Catarina, Florianópolis, 1998. 226 p.

FERRAZ, L.. **The care provided to the child by the family and indigenous community in the perception of health professionals**. Dissertation (Master in Nursing), Federal University of Santa Catarina, Florianópolis, 2010.

FOLLÉR, M.-L. Intermedicality: the contact zone created by indigenous peoples and health professionals. In: LANGDON, E. J.; GARNELO, L. (Org.). **Indigenous peoples' health**: reflections on participatory anthropology. Rio de Janeiro: ContraCapa/ABA, 2004. pp. 129-148.

GARCIA, S. C. P. **Diabetes and hypertension among Kaingang indigenous people from Aldeia Sede, TIX**: self-care practices in a context of intermedicality. Dissertation (Master's), Graduate Program in Social Anthropology, Federal University of Santa Catarina, Florianópolis, 2010.

GARNELO, L.; MACEDO, G.; BRANDÃO, L. C. **Os povos indígenas e a construção das políticas de saúde no Brasil.** Brasília: Panamerican Health Organization, 2003.

GEERTZ, C. **A interpretação das culturas**. Rio de Janeiro: Guanabara Koogan Publishers, 1978.

HAVERROTH, M.. **Kaingang an ethnobotanical study**: the use and classification of plants in the Xapecó Indigenous Area (West of SC). Dissertation (Master's Degree in Social Anthropology), Federal University of Santa Catarina, 1997.

IDS/SSL/CEBRAP. Consórcio IDS-SSL-CEBRAP (Institute of Development Studies/Health Without Limits/Brazilian Center for Analysis and Planning). **Diagnóstico Situacional do Subsistema de Saúde Indígena**. Relatório Inicial (revised). Brasília, 2009.

LANGDON, E. J.; DIEHL, E. E. Participação e autonomia nos espaços interculturais de Saúde Indígena: reflexões a partir do sul do Brasil. **Saúde e Sociedade**, v. 16, n. 2, pp. 19-36, 2007.

LANGDON, E. J.; DIEHL, E. E.; WIIK, F. B.; DIAS-SCOPEL, R. P. The participation of indigenous health agents in health care services: the experience in Santa Catarina, Brazil. **Cadernos de Saúde Pública**, Rio de Janeiro, v. 22, n. 12, dez. 2006. Available at: <http://www.scielo.br/scielo.php?script=sci_arttext&pid=S0102-311X2006001200013&lng=en&nrm=iso>. Accessed on: 19 May 2010.

LEININGER, M. M. **Culture care Diversity & Universality**: A Theory of Nursing. New York: National League for Nursing Press, 1991.

MARINHO, G. L.; OTT, A. T. **Agentes indígenas de saúde de Rondônia: um estudo etnográfico** (Preliminary Report). Programa Institucional de Bolsas de Iniciação Científica (Pibic), Universidade de Rondônia/Centro de Estudos de Saúde Indígena de Rondônia (Cesir)/CNPq, 2007. 32 p.

MENDONÇA, S. B. M. O Agente Indígena de Saúde do Parque vigilância à saúde indígena do Xingu: reflexões. In: BARUZZZI, R.; JUNQUEIRA, C. (Org.). **Indigenous Park of Xingu: health, culture and history**. São Paulo: Unifesp/Terra Virgem, 2005. pp. 227-246.

MOROSINI, M. V. G. C.; CORBO, A. D'. (Org.). **Modelos de atenção e a saúde da família**. Rio de Janeiro: EPSJV/Fiocruz, 2007.

MOTA, L. T.; NOELLI, F. S.; T.OMMASINO, K. (Org.). **URI e Wãxi**: estudos interdisciplinares dos Kaingang. Londrina: UEL, 2000. 377 p.

MOTA, R. R. A; DAVID, H. M. S. L. The increasing schooling of the community health agent: an induction of the work process? **Trabalho, Educação e Saúde**, Rio de Janeiro, v. 8 n. 2, pp. 229-248, jul./out. 2010.

NACKE, A.; RENK, A.; PIOVEZANA, L.; BLOEMER, N. M. S. **Os Kaingang no Oeste Catarinense**. Chapecó, SC: Argos, 2007. 158 p.

NIMUENDAJÚ, C. **Etnografia e indigenismo**: sobre os Kaingang, os Ofaié-Xavante e os índios do Pará. Campinas: Unicamp, 1993.

NOELLI, F. et al. **Bibliografia Kaingáing**: referências sobre um povo Jê no sul do Brasil. Londrina: UEL, 1998.

NOTZOLD, A. L. V. (Org.). **The Kaingáng life cycle**. Florianópolis: University Press of UFSC, 2004.

NOVO, M. P. **Os agentes indígenas de saúde do Alto Xingu**. Dissertation (Master's Degree), Graduate Program in Social Anthropology, Universidade Federal de São Carlos, SP, 2008.

NOVO, M. P. **Os agentes indígenas de saúde do Alto Xingu**. Brasília: ABA, 2010.

NUNES, M. O. et al. O agente comunitário de saúde: construção da identidade desse personagem híbrido e polifônico. **Cadernos de Saúde Pública**, Rio de Janeiro, v. 18, n. 6, dez. 2002. Available at: <http://www. scielosp. org/scielo. php?script=sci_arttext&pid=S0102- 311X2002000600018&lng=en&nrm=iso>. Accessed on: 2 Jun. 2011.

OLIVEIRA, L. S. S. O agente indígena de saúde do Parque Indígena do Xingu:

perspectivas de formação e trabalho. In: BARUZZZI, R. G.; JUNQUEIRA, C. (Org.). **Indigenous Park of Xingu**: health, culture and history. São Paulo: Terra Virgem, 2005.

OLIVEIRA, M. C. **Curador Kaingang e a recriação de suas práticas**: estudo de caso na aldeia Xapecó. Dissertation (Master's Degree in Social Anthropology), Universidade Federal de Santa Catarina, Florianópolis, 1996.

OLIVEIRA, P. H. **Comida forte e comida fraca**: alimentação e fabricação dos corpos entre os Kaingang da Terra Indígena Xapecó. 2009. Dissertation (Master's in Anthropology), Federal University of Santa Catarina, Florianópolis, 2010.

PEDUZZI, M.; ANSELMI, M. L. (Coord.). **Final research report**: evaluation of the impact of Profae on the quality of health services. Brasil. Ministério da Saúde. São Paulo, 2004.

PORTELA, S. C. **Diabetes and hypertension among Kaingang indigenous people from the Sede village, TIX**: practice of self-care in a context of intermedicality. Dissertation (Master's in Social Anthropology), Federal University of Santa Catarina, Florianópolis, 2010.

RIBEIRO, M. I. L. C.; PEDRÃO, L. J. Relacionamento interpessoal no nível médio de enfermagem. **Revista Brasileira de Enfermagem**, v. 58, n. 3, 2005. Available at: <http://www.scielo.br/scielo.php?script=sci_arttext&pid=S0034-71672005000300011&lng=en&nrm=iso>. Accessed on: 8 Nov. 2009.

ROCHA, C. C. **Adoecer e curar:** processos da sociabilidade Kaingang. 2005. Dissertation (Master's in Social Anthropology), Universidade Federal de Santa Catarina, Florianópolis, 2005.

ROCHA, S. M. M; ALMEIDA, M. C. P. O processo de trabalho da enfermagem em saúde coletiva e a interdisciplinariedade. **Revista Latino-americana de Enfermagem**, v. 8, n. 6, pp. 96-101, dec. 2000.

ROSA, R. R. G. **"Os Kujá são diferentes"**: um estudo etnológico do complexo xamânico dos Kaingang da Terra Indígena Votouro. 2005. 416f. Thesis (Doctorate in Social Anthropology), Federal University of Rio Grande do Sul, Porto Alegre, 2005.

SANTOS, S. C. **Indigenismo e expansão capitalista**: faces da agonia Kaingang. Florianópolis: UFSC, 1979.

SCHIMITH, M. D.; LIMA, M. A. D. S. Acolhimento e vínculo em uma equipe do Programa Saúde da Família. **Cadernos de Saúde Pública**, Rio de Janeiro, v.

20, n. 6, dez. 2004. Available at:
<http:// www. scielosp. org/scielo. php? script=sci_arttext&pid=S0102-311X2004000600005&lng=en&nrm=iso>. Accessed on: 14 Jun. 2011.

SHIMIZU, H. E.; DYTZ, J. L. G.; LIMA, M. G.; MOURA, A. S. A prática do auxiliar de enfemagem do Programa Saúde da Família.
Revista Latino-Americana de Enfermagem, v. 12, n. 5, pp. 713-720, sep./out. 2004.

SILVA, J. A.; DALMASO, A. S.W. O agente comunitário de saúde e suas atribuições: os desafios para os processos de formação de recursos humanos em saúde. **Interface Journal**, v. 6, n. 10, pp. 75-96, feb. 2002.

SIMIEMA, J. Em que abrigos se alojarão? In: MOTA, L. T.; NOELLI, F. S.; TOMMASINO, K. (Org.). **URI e Wãxi**: estudos interdisciplinares dos Kaingang. Londrina: UEL, 2000.

SOUSA, M. C.; SCATENA, J. H. G.; SANTOS, R. V. O Sistema de Informação da Atenção à Saúde Indígena (SIASI): criação, estrutura e funcionamento. **Cadernos de Saúde Pública**, v. 23, n. 4, pp. 853-861, abr. 2007. Available at:
<http:// www.scielo.br/scielo. php?script=sci_arttext&pid=S0102-311X2007000400013&lng=pt&nrm=iso>. Accessed: 27 Jun. 2011.

TOMMASINO, K.; FERNANDES, R.C. Kaingang. 2001. Available at:
<http://pib.socioambiental.org/pt/povo/kaingang/286>. Accessed on: 5 Oct. 2010.

VEIGA, J. **Organização social e cosmovisão Kaingang**: uma introdução ao parentesco, casamento e nominação em uma sociedade Jê meridional.1994. Dissertation (Master's in Anthropology)- Programa de Pós Graduação em Antropologia Social, Universiadade de Campinas, Unicamp, Campinas, 1994.

WALDOW et al. Cuidar/cuidado: o domínio unificador da enfermagem. In: WALDOW, V. R. et al. **Maneiras de cuidar, maneiras de ensinar**: a enfermagem entre a escola e a prática profissional. Porto Alegre: Artes médicas, 1995.

WENDHAUSEN, Á. L. P.; RIVERA, S. O cuidado de si como princípio ético do trabalho em enfermagem. **Texto & Contexto Enfermagem**, Florianópolis, v. 14, n. 1, mar. 2005. Available at:
<http://www.scielo.br/scielo.php?script=sci_arttext&pid=S0104-07072005000100015&lng=en&nrm=iso>. Accessed on: 16 Jun. 2011.

WHO. Word Health Organization. Alma-Ata Declaration. In: **International**

conference on primary health care, WHO, 1978. Available at:
<http://www.who.int/publications/almaata_declaration_en.pdf>. Accessed on:
22 May 2011.

APPENDIX

APPENDIX 1

**Interview schedule for nursing technician/nursing assistant (interview both
indigenous and non-indigenous people)**

1. Name:
2. Sex:
3. Education (years completed):
4. Name and place of the Nursing Technician/Auxiliary Course you
   attended:
5. When he graduated as a nursing technician/auxiliary:
6. Was the technical/nursing assistant course free or
   paid? If paid, who paid?
7. How long did the Nursing Technician/Auxiliary Course last? Ask for
   the total workload.
8. How the workload was distributed (theoretical lessons; practical
   lessons; morning, afternoon and/or evening).
9. How long have you worked as a nursing technician/auxiliary:
10. Have you ever worked as a nursing technician/auxiliary in another
    indigenous area? If yes, ask where and what he was doing.
11. Have you ever worked as a nursing technician/auxiliary outside the

area

    indigenous? If yes, ask where and what he was doing.
12. Currently employed by whom:
13. Position currently held in the health team:
14. How was the choice for this position?

15. Time in current position:

16. Salary: request in terms of number of minimum wages.

17. Have you had other positions in the village health team? If yes, which ones and for how long. Find out if you have been an Agent

Indigenous Health (ISA). If you have been an ISA, ask them to compare what they did as an ISA and what they do now, pointing out positive and negative aspects.

18. What is your current role/role in the health team? Ask them to describe all the activities/tasks they carry out, emphasizing the tasks they do alone and those they carry out with other team members.

19. What are the facilities to carry out these tasks?

20. What are the difficulties in carrying out these tasks?

21. Do you think your role in the health team should be different? If yes, ask to explain what and how it should be different.

22. Ask them to make an evaluation of their work, commenting on their relationship with the health team (integration, team building, etc.).

23. Ask them to make an evaluation of their work, commenting on their relationship with the community (what is good/bad and what should be changed to improve).

At the end, ask them to show any and all material made available by the Technical/Nursing Assistant Course (diploma, folder, course structure, handouts, etc.).
Socio-demographic data and other education/training:

1. Marital status:

2. Number of children: ask to give the ages of each child and how many still depend on him/her.

3. How many and which people live in the house:

4. Is the house yours?

5. kinship/relationship with leaders: ask about kinship/relationship with chieftain, captain, post chief, municipal administrators, etc.

6. Religion/Church you attend.

7. In the case of indigenous, what ethnicity?

8. Do you speak the language?

9. Besides the Nursing Technician/Auxiliary Course, what other training and capacity-building courses have you taken? Ask them to describe each one, stating:

    a. Content;

    b. who promoted it;

    c. year in which it took place;

    d. duration;

    e. location;

    f. what the positive and negative aspects of each are.

If possible, ask to show the certificate(s) and materials made available by the Training Courses.

APPENDIX 2

Interview script for coordinators and/or teachers of technical/nursing assistant courses

1. Sex:

2. Age:

3. Professional activity:

4. Training:

5. Course Binding (name of the institution promoting the Course):

6. Course Name:

7. Public or private course:

8. If private, what is the cost to the student?

9. How often does this course take place?

10. What is the workload?

11. How are the course hours distributed in the week?

12. What methodology is used?

13. What is the scope of the Course?

14. How was the course publicised?

15. Are there specific courses for indigenous people? If yes, which ones and how many have already been held?

16. How many were enrolled and how many graduated? Specify Indigenous people.

17. Where were the students from?

18. Were there many drop-outs? Why have there been many drop-outs?

19. In the case of indigenous people, how do you evaluate their participation in the Course?

Request at the end all and any material used in the Course (promotional folder, Course structure, handouts, etc.).

APPENDIX 3

Interview schedule for other members of the Multidisciplinary Indigenous Health Team (EMSI)

1. Name:

2. Sex:

3. Education (years completed):

4. Year, institution and place where you graduated (ask in relation to the highest degree):

5. How long have you worked in this profession (specify: doctor, dentist, nurse, nutritionist, etc.)?

6. Have you ever worked in another indigenous area? If yes, ask where and what he did.

7. How long have you worked in this indigenous area?

8. Currently employed by whom:

9. Position currently held in the health team:

10. How was the choice for this position?

11. Time in current position:

12. Salary: request in terms of number of minimum wages.

13. Have you had other positions in the village health team? If yes, which and for how long.

14. How do you work with the nursing technician/assistant? Ask them to describe the activities/tasks they perform together with the nursing technician/assistant.

15. Ask them to comment on the facilities and difficulties of the working relationship with the nursing technician/auxiliary, seeking to

compare when the nursing technician/auxiliary is indigenous or not.

16. Should the role/function of the nursing technician/auxiliary in the health team be different? If yes, ask to explain what and how it should be different.

APPENDIX 4

Informed Consent Form (ICF)

Nursing technicians/assistants

I am Helga Follmann, a Master's student in the Postgraduate Programme in Public Health, and you are being invited to take part in our research on the *Insertion of the Indigenous Nursing Technician/Auxiliary on Kaingáng Indigenous Land (Santa Catarina): An Analysis On Their Role In The Indigenous Health Care Model* and this research aims to analyse the role of the indigenous nursing technician and assistant in their community, to verify the students who took the technical course, how they feel about their work, how the community feels about the work of indigenous nursing technicians/auxiliaries and how the health teams feel about working with the indigenous nursing technician health professional, with the aim of analysing how the training courses and training of nursing technicians/auxiliaries do to adapt in intercultural situations.

I will identify the indigenous nursing technicians/assistants working in the Xapecó Indigenous Land and the actions that they should take, considering the organization of the health services and the view of the indigenous nursing technicians/assistants themselves, as well as the difficulties they face. To do this, I will accompany you [indigenous technicians/nursing assistants] in your activities.

For the development of the research, visits will be made to the Health Posts where you attend and the monitoring of the

indigenous nursing technicians/assistants in their functions. In these visits, I will interview you with questions and I will also try to talk about the activities of the indigenous nursing technician/auxiliary in your community, how the health team sees the work of this professional and how the community feels in relation to this professional, among other issues related to the theme and that you may find important. With you, the indigenous nurse technician/auxiliary in your community, I will try to talk about issues related to your work. In these interviews and conversations, the tape recorder and/or camera may be used. I make it clear that these procedures are not aggressive or harmful to your life and that the tape recorder and/or the camera will only be used if you give your permission.

Any questions you have about the work or if you want to withdraw from the research (no harm to you) you can contact me Helga Follmann, personally at the address: Rua João Saturnino Ouriques, 712, São José -SC CEP 88101-330 or by email: enfermeirahelga@gmail.com, or by phone (48) 8454-5887 or with the project coordinator, Prof.[1] Eliana E. Diehl at the following address: Departamento de Ciências Farmacêuticas, Centro de Ciências da Saúde, Universidade Federal de Santa Catarina, Campus Universitário, Trindade, Florianópolis, SC - CEP 88040-900; Fone: 48-3331-9350 ou 48-3331-5077.

If you agree to participate, I can state that the information you provide will be kept confidential, ensuring your privacy regarding the confidential data involved in the research.

I also guarantee that there is no expense to you. The results of the research will be made public, whether favourable or unfavourable, and the data collected will be used for writing articles and other dissemination materials such as books, reports, posters, etc. The communities will receive a copy of all the material produced.

After reading this Statement, I would like to know if you accept to participate in the research. If you accept, I request that you sign the Consent Form below.

A. PROJECT IDENTIFICATION

"The Insertion of the Indigenous Nursing Technician/Auxiliary in Kaingáng Indigenous Land (Santa Catarina): An Analysis of Their Role in the Indigenous Health Care Model"

Master's researcher: Helga Follmann

Coordinator: Profa. Eliana Elisabeth Diehl

B. OPINIONS ON ETHICAL ASPECTS:

Ethics Committee in Research with Human Beings/UFSC: 626/2010

National Research Ethics Committee (Conep): 0540/2010

FREE AND INFORMED CONSENT FORM[1]

I declare that I was informed about all the procedures of the research and that I received, in a clear and objective way, all the explanations about the project. I understand that the information provided will be kept confidential, ensuring my privacy as to the confidential data involved in the research. I was also informed that there are no expenses for me.

I declare that I have been informed that I can withdraw from the study at any time.

....of ....2010.

Village:...

Name by

in full: ....Signature:

ID (where applicable):

Name and signature of witness (Indian who cannot read or write): ....

APPENDIX 5

Informed Consent Form (ICF)

Teachers and coordinators

I am Helga Follmann, a Master's student in the Postgraduate Programme in Public Health, and you are being invited to participate in our research project about ***The Insertion of the Indigenous Nursing Technician/Auxiliary on Kaingáng Indigenous Land (Santa Catarina): An Analysis On Their Role In The Indigenous Health Care Model*** and this research aims to analyse the role of the indigenous nursing technician and assistant in their community, to verify the students who took the technical course, how they feel about their work, how the community feels about the work of indigenous nursing technicians/auxiliaries and how the health teams feel about working with the indigenous nursing technician health professional, with the aim of analysing how the training courses and training of nursing technicians/auxiliaries do to adapt in intercultural situations.

I also have the objective of identifying: the Kaingáng students who started and finished courses for nursing technicians or assistants, with emphasis on the "Pioneer Project" of the UFSC held in 2001; the profile of the indigenous professional who finished courses for nursing technicians or assistants, with emphasis on the "Pioneer Project" of the UFSC held in 2001; the institutional strategies of training for nursing technicians or assistants; the activities of the indigenous nursing technician/auxiliary in their community.

For the development of the research, interviews will be conducted with teachers and coordinators of the technical/nursing assistant course(s) of the institutions that provided training for indigenous professionals. In these interviews and conversations, the tape recorder and/or camera may be used. I make it clear that these procedures are not aggressive or harmful to your life and that the tape recorder and/or the camera will only be used if you give your permission.

Any questions you have about the work or if you want to withdraw from the research (no harm to you) you can contact me Helga Follmann, personally at the address: Rua João Saturnino Ouriques, 712, São José -SC CEP 88101-330 or by email: enfermeirahelga@gmail.com, or by phone (48) 8454-5887 or with the project coordinator, Prof.[1] Eliana E. Diehl at the following address: Departamento de Ciências Farmacêuticas, Centro de Ciências da Saúde, Universidade Federal de Santa Catarina, Campus Universitário, Trindade, Florianópolis, SC - CEP 88040-900; Fone: 48-3331-9350 ou 48-3331-5077.

If you agree to participate, I can assure you that the information you provide will be kept confidential, ensuring your privacy regarding the confidential data involved in the research. I can also assure you that there will be no expense to you. The results of the research will be made public, whether favourable or unfavourable, and the data collected will be used for writing articles and other dissemination materials such as books, reports, posters, etc. The communities will receive a copy of all the material produced.

After reading this Statement, I would like to know if you accept to participate in the research. If you accept, I request that you sign the Consent Form below.

APPENDIX 6

Informed Consent Form (ICF)

Multidisciplinary Health Team

I am Helga Follmann, a Master's student in the Postgraduate Programme in Public Health, and you are being invited to participate in our research project about ***The Insertion of the Indigenous Nursing Technician/Auxiliary on Kaingáng Indigenous Land (Santa Catarina): An Analysis On Their Role In The Indigenous Health Care Model*** and this research aims to analyse the role of the indigenous nursing technician and assistant in their community, to verify the students who took the technical course, how they feel about their work, how the community feels about the work of indigenous nursing technicians/auxiliaries and how the health teams feel about working with the indigenous nursing technician health professional, with the aim of analysing how the training courses and training of nursing technicians/auxiliaries do to adapt in intercultural situations.

I also aim to identify the activities of the indigenous nursing technician/auxiliary in your community and how you, an integral part of the multidisciplinary indigenous health team, feel about the work of this professional.

For the development of the research, interviews and observation of the team's health professionals working in the indigenous area will be carried out. In these interviews and conversations, a tape recorder may be used

and/or the camera. I make it clear that these procedures are not aggressive or harmful to your life and that the recorder and/or the camera will only be used if you give your permission.

Any questions you have about the work or if you want to withdraw from the research (no harm to you) you can contact me Helga Follmann, personally at the address: Rua João Saturnino Ouriques, 712, São José -SC CEP 88101-330 or by email: enfermeirahelga@gmail.com, or by phone (48) 8454-5887 or with the project coordinator, Prof.[1] Eliana E. Diehl at the following address: Departamento de Ciências Farmacêuticas, Centro de Ciências da Saúde, Universidade Federal de Santa Catarina, Campus Universitário, Trindade, Florianópolis, SC - CEP 88040-900; Fone: 48-3331-9350 ou 48-3331-5077.

If you agree to participate, I can assure you that the information you provide will be kept confidential, ensuring your privacy regarding the confidential data involved in the research. I can also assure you that there will be no expense to you. The results of the research will be made public, whether favourable or unfavourable, and the data collected will be used for writing articles and other dissemination materials such as books, reports, posters, etc. The communities will receive a copy of all the material produced.

After reading this Statement, I would like to know if you accept to participate in the research. If you accept, I request that you sign the Consent Form below.

ANNEX

ANNEX 1

Opinion of the Ethics Committee of the Federal University of Santa Catarina

MINISTÉRIO DA SAÚDE
Conselho Nacional de Saúde
Comissão Nacional de Ética em Pesquisa - CONEP

FOLHA DE ROSTO PARA PESQUISA ENVOLVENDO SERES HUMANOS　　**FR - 349005**

Projeto de Pesquisa
A inserção do técnico/auxiliar indígena de enfermagem em Terra Indígena Kaingáng (Santa Catarina): uma análise sobre o seu papel no modelo de atenção à saúde indígena

Área de Conhecimento	Grupo	Nível
4.00 - Ciências da Saúde - 4.06 - Saúde Coletiva - Nenhum	Grupo I	Não se aplica

Área(s) Temática(s) Especial(s)	Fase
Populações Indígenas	Não se Aplica

Unitermos
Saúde Indígena, Auxiliares de Enfermagem, Índios Sul-Americanos

Sujeitos na Pesquisa			
Nº de Sujeitos no Centro	Total Brasil	Nº de Sujeitos Total	Grupos Especiais
50	50	50	

Placebo	Medicamentos HIV / AIDS	Wash-out	Sem Tratamento Específico	Banco de Materiais Biológicos
NÃO	NÃO	NÃO	NÃO	NÃO

Pesquisador Responsável

Pesquisador Responsável	CPF	Identidade
Eliana Elisabeth Diehl	405.276.630-34	39402932

Área de Especialização	Maior Titulação	Nacionalidade
Saúde Pública	Doutorado	brasileira

Endereço	Bairro	Cidade
Depto de Ciências Farmacêuticas, UFSC	Trindade	Florianópolis - SC

Código Postal	Telefone	Fax	Email
88040-900	48-3721-9350 /	48-3721-9542	ELIANADIEHL@HOTMAIL.COM

Termo de Compromisso

Declaro que conheço e cumprirei os requisitos da Res. CNS 196/96 e suas complementares. Comprometo-me a utilizar os materiais e dados coletados exclusivamente para os fins previstos no protocolo e publicar os resultados sejam eles favoráveis ou não.
Aceito as responsabilidades pela condução científica do projeto acima.

Data: 14 / 06 / 2010　　　　　　　　　　Assinatura

Instituição Onde Será Realizado

Nome	CNPJ	Nacional/Internacional
Universidade Federal de Santa Catarina - UFSC	83.899.525/0001-82	Nacional

Unidade/Órgão	Participação Estrangeira	Projeto Multicêntrico
Departamento de Ciências Farmacêuticas	NÃO	NÃO

Endereço	Bairro	Cidade
Campus Universitário Reitor João David Ferreira Lima	Trindade	Florianópolis - SC

Código Postal	Telefone	Fax	Email
88040-900	48 3319206	48 3319599	cep@reitoria.ufsc.br

Termo de Compromisso

Declaro que conheço e cumprirei os requisitos da Res. CNS 196/96 e suas complementares e como esta instituição tem condições para o desenvolvimento deste projeto, autorizo sua execução.

Nome: ROSANE MARIA BUDAL
Data: 14 / 06 / 2010　　　　　　　　　Assinatura:
Prof.ª Drª Rosane Maria Budal
Chefe do CIF/CCS/UFSC

O Projeto deverá ser entregue no CEP em até 30 dias a partir de 14/06/2010. Não ocorrendo a entrega nesse prazo esta Folha de Rosto será INVALIDADA.

○Voltar　　　　　　　　　IMPRIMIR

ANNEX 2

Authorization from the National Research Ethics Committee (Conep)

MINISTÉRIO DA SAÚDE
Conselho Nacional de Saúde

OFÍCIO Nº. 3005/10/CONEP/CNS/MS

Brasília-DF, 29 de setembro de 2010.

Assunto: *"Encaminhamento de Parecer".*

Senhor (a) Coordenador (a),

1.   Encaminhamos, em anexo, o (s) Parecer (es) nº **0540/2010, referente ao Protocolo de Pesquisa Registro CONEP nº 16.034** da Comissão Nacional de Ética em Pesquisa – CONEP, referente(s) a (os) projeto(s) de pesquisa acompanhada(s) por esse Comitê.

Atenciosamente,

ROZÂNGELA FERNANDES CAMAPUM
SECRETÁRIA-EXECUTIVA DO
CONSELHO NACIONAL DE SAÚDE

Ao Senhor (a) Washington Portela de Souza
Coordenador (a) do Comitê de Ética em Pesquisas
Universidade Federal de Santa Catarina - UFSC
Campus Universitário - Trindade
Florianópolis SC
Cep: 88.040-900

SI/lc

Esplanada dos Ministérios Bloco "G" – Edifício Anexo, Ala "B" – 1º andar, Sala 104 – 70058-900 – Brasília, DF
Telefones: (061) 3226-8603 / 3225-8672 – Fax: (061) 3315-2414 / 3315-2472 – e-mail: cns@saude.gov.br

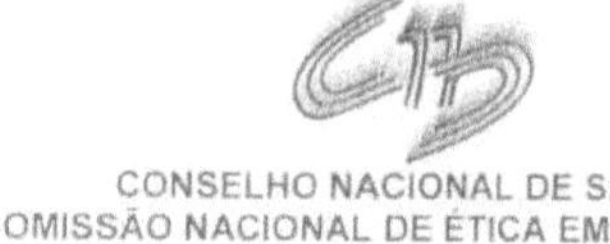

CONSELHO NACIONAL DE SAÚDE
COMISSÃO NACIONAL DE ÉTICA EM PESQUISA

PARECER Nº 540/2010

Registro CONEP 16034 (Este nº deve ser citado nas correspondências referentes a este projeto)

CAAE – 0127.0.242.000-10   Processo nº 25000.116333/2010-61

Projeto de Pesquisa: *"A inserção do técnico/auxiliar indígena de enfermagem em Terra Indígena Kaingáng (Santa Catarina): uma análise sobre o seu papel no modelo de atenção à saúde indígena"*

Pesquisador Responsável: Eliana Elisabeth Diehl

Instituição: Universidade Federal de Santa Catarina **(CENTRO ÚNICO)**

CEP de origem: da instituição (CEPSH/CEUA)

Área Temática Especial: Populações Indígenas

Patrocinador: não especificado.

Sumário geral do protocolo

No contexto da saúde indígena, se observa o aumento gradativo de indígenas e a busca e formação de profissionais que atuem como técnicos ou auxiliares de enfermagem em comunidades indígenas. Na Equipe Multidisciplinar de Atenção Básica à Saúde Indígena (EMSI), o técnico/auxiliar de enfermagem é o profissional que tem maior contato com a população depois do agente indígena de saúde (AIS), tendo atividades mais complexas que o AIS e em alguns casos assumindo a coordenação local do serviço. Entretanto, trabalhos recentes mostram que, geralmente, os membros da EMSI encontram-se despreparados para lidar com as diferentes culturas com as quais interagem no processo de trabalho nas comunidades indígenas. Pesquisas anteriores evidenciaram que a atenção diferenciada está longe de tornar-se realidade e apontam que uma das principais dificuldades está na falta de formação e capacitação dos profissionais de saúde para atuar em contextos interétnicos e, apesar do Subsistema de atenção à saúde indígena estar em funcionamento desde 1999, são raros estudos sobre o papel dos profissionais de saúde e a adequação de cursos de formação e capacitação para a atuação em situações interculturais. Tais pesquisas são essenciais para subsidiar as políticas públicas, a formação de recursos humanos para atuação em contextos interculturais e, por consequência, a melhoria da qualidade dos serviços.

O objetivo geral do projeto é 'analisar o papel do técnico e auxiliar indígena de enfermagem, focalizando a sua formação e atuação na equipe multiprofissional de saúde indígena (EMSI)'. Os objetivos específicos são: 1-Identificar os alunos Kaingáng que iniciaram e finalizaram Cursos para técnico ou auxiliar de enfermagem, com ênfase para o "Projeto Pioneiro" da UFSC realizado em 2001; 2- Identificar o perfil do profissional indígena que concluiu Cursos para técnico ou auxiliar de enfermagem, com ênfase para o "Projeto Pioneiro" da UFSC realizado em 2001; 3-Identificar as estratégias institucionais de capacitação para técnico ou auxiliar de enfermagem; 4-Identificar as atividades do técnico/auxiliar indígena de enfermagem em sua comunidade; 5-Analisar a autopercepção sobre o papel e inserção na Equipe Multiprofissional de Saúde Indígena; 6- Analisar a percepção da Equipe Multiprofissional de Saúde Indígena sobre o papel do técnico e auxiliar indígena de enfermagem; 7- Analisar a percepção da comunidade sobre o papel do técnico e auxiliar indígena de enfermagem.

1/4   db/ lc

94

O desenho da pesquisa agrega (a) pesquisa documental/bibliográfica junto aos Cursos de formação para técnico e auxiliar de enfermagem e se necessário junto à Fundação Nacional de Saúde (FUNASA), aos Pólos-Base e às Secretarias Municipais de Saúde da região abrangida pelo Distrito Sanitário Especial Indígena Interior Sul, o qual pertence a Terra Indígena Xapecó; (b) aplicação de questionário sócio-econômico aos técnicos e auxiliares de enfermagem; (c) entrevistas com coordenadores e/ou professores de Cursos profissionalizantes de técnico e auxiliar de enfermagem ("Projeto Pioneiro" da UFSC, Escolas Técnicas do SUS e Cursos privados) (d) Pesquisas de Campo e observação participante. Para este fim, o pesquisador permanecerá em campo pelo período máximo de 150 dias corridos ou com intervalos entre eles, dependendo da necessidade. As atividades dos técnicos e auxiliares de enfermagem (indígenas e não indígenas) e do restante da Equipe serão acompanhadas, bem como eles serão entrevistados acerca do papel dos técnicos e auxiliares indígenas de enfermagem (autopercepção e percepção da EMSI). Ainda será conduzida observação participante durante as interações entre os profissionais e os usuários dos serviços de saúde. Esses usuários poderão ser entrevistados visando investigar a percepção sobre o papel do técnico e auxiliar indígena de enfermagem.

Com relação a inclusão e exclusão dos participantes no estudo, tem-se que: os indivíduos serão incluídos na pesquisa caso recebam o convite e concordem com a pesquisa e assinatura do Termo de Consentimento Livre e Esclarecido e deixarão de participar a qualquer momento da pesquisa, sem danos diretos ou indiretos.

No que diz respeito aos riscos, a pesquisadora aponta que, dado o caráter etnográfico da pesquisa "não há riscos que ameacem a vida ou o bem-estar dos indivíduos envolvidos durante o trabalho de campo. Os dados gerados poderão servir como subsídios para o planejamento e implementação de ações e serviços de saúde voltados às comunidades indígenas. Todos os procedimentos para a coleta dos dados não são invasivos sob o aspecto físico e se fará previamente todos os esclarecimentos necessários a cada indivíduo que participar da pesquisa, conforme Termo de Consentimento Livre e Esclarecido em anexo. O gravador de voz somente será utilizado após consentimento dos informantes.)" (página 19, numeração do CEP).

Com relação aos benefícios não há registro de trabalhos que contemplem os técnicos/auxiliares indígenas de enfermagem, essa pesquisa permitirá uma avaliação dos papéis desses profissionais no Subsistema de atenção à saúde indígena. A análise das estratégias institucionais de capacitação desses profissionais fornecerá subsídios para adequar a sua formação visando atuação em contextos étnicos específicos. Esses dois aspectos analisados têm potencial contribuição para a melhoria da qualidade dos serviços prestados aos povos indígenas. Ao final, os resultados da pesquisa deverão ser divulgados através de relatórios, artigos, participação em eventos científicos e em eventos promovidos pela sociedade organizada (por exemplo, Conselho Distrital de Saúde Indígena e Comissão Intersetorial de Saúde Indígena), entre outras atividades. Os resultados serão divulgados às comunidades que geraram os dados, às instituições envolvidas na prestação de serviços de saúde aos índios em Santa Catarina e à FUNASA.

Local de realização

Trata-se de um projeto nacional e unicêntrico. O total de sujeitos de pesquisa para cada sub-grupo estudado não foi especificado, embora conste na Folha de Rosto (página 1, numeração do CEP) o total de 50 pessoas. A pesquisa documental/bibliográfica será realizada junto aos Cursos de formação para técnico e auxiliar de enfermagem e se necessário junto à Fundação Nacional de Saúde (FUNASA), aos Pólos-Base e às Secretarias Municipais de Saúde da região abrangida pelo Distrito Sanitário Especial Indígena Interior Sul, o qual pertence a Terra Indígena Xapecó. A pesquisa de campo propriamente dita será realizada na Terra Indígena Xapecó em quatro aldeias, quais sejam aldeias Sede, Pinhalzinho e Fazenda São José (localizadas geograficamente no município de Ipuaçu) e aldeia Paiol de Barro (localizada no município de Entre Rios).

Apresentação do protocolo

A folha de rosto foi apresentada na página 01 (numeração do CEP), com a assinatura da pesquisadora responsável pela instituição, no entanto, a versão apresentada impressa está muito clara e pouco legível. Nas páginas 02 a 07 foi encaminhada a cópia de formulário com dados do protocolo. O cronograma é apresentado tanto na página 20, quanto na página 33 (numeração do CEP) e o orçamento é apresentado tanto na página 21, quanto na página 31 (numeração do CEP) com valor bruto de R$ 6000,00 envolvendo gastos com material de consumo, despesas de correio e diárias. O TCLE a ser apresentado aos técnicos/auxiliares de enfermagem é apresentado na página 08 (numeração do CEP). O parecer consubstanciado é apresentado nas páginas 40 a 42 e assinado pelo coordenador do CEP. Os instrumentos para coleta de dados apresentados são: (1) Roteiro de entrevistas para outros membros da equipe multidisciplinar de saúde indígena (páginas 24 e 25, numeração do CEP), (2) e Roteiro de entrevistas para técnicos e auxiliares de enfermagem (páginas 26 a 28, numeração do CEP), (3) Roteiro de entrevistas para coordenadores e/ou professores de curso técnico /auxiliar de Enfermagem (página 29, numeração do CEP) E (4) Roteiro de entrevista para a comunidade (página 30, numeração do CEP). A autorização da Funasa é apresentada nas páginas 34 e 35 (numeração do CEP) e carta de autorização do cacique da Terra indígena Xapecó na página 39 (numeração do CEP). Os endereços para acesso ao curículos *lattes* das pesquisadoras principais são apresentado na página 02 (numeração do CEP).

Comentários/Considerações

1. Solicita-se ao pesquisador informar o número de sujeitos de pesquisa que farão parte do projeto, uma vez que o universo da pesquisa não foi bem delimitado;
2. Com relação ao título do projeto: *"A inserção do técnico/auxiliar indígena de enfermagem em Terra indígena Kaingáng (Santa Catarina), uma análise sobre o seu papel no modelo de atenção à saúde indígena"*, é feita menção à terra indígena *"Kaingáng"*, no entanto, não é feita a especificação em quais aldeias de fato será realizada a pesquisa, quais sejam: Aldeia sede, Pinhalzinho, Fazenda São José e Paiol de Barro. Além disso, por vezes a pesquisadora faz menção à pesquisa fazendo menção ao local de realização, como sendo "Terra indígena Kaingáng" e por vezes à "Terra indígena Xapecó". Ainda que seja feita nota de rodapé na página 15 (numeração do CEP), solicita-se uniformizar a designação ao local de realização em todo protocolo.
3. Com relação aos riscos/benefícios da pesquisa, segundo Resolução CNS 196/96, item V: "Considera-se que toda pesquisa envolvendo seres humanos envolve risco. O dano eventual poderá ser imediato ou tardio, comprometendo o indivíduo ou a coletividade". Nesses termos, o pesquisador se equivoca ao afirmar: (a) "Toda a parte operacional da pesquisa é de natureza etnográfica, com coleta de informações que não envolvem intervenções invasivas ou que denotem riscos à integridade física, psíquica/emocional, moral, social e cultural dos indivíduos e dos grupos. Dadas as características da pesquisa, não há a possibilidade de qualquer dano ambiental ou nutricional." (pág. 03, numeração do CEP) e novamente, ao afirmar: "Não há riscos que ameacem a vida ou o bem-estar dos indivíduos" (Pág. 41, numeração do CEP). Solicita-se adequação do texto.
4. Em relação ao Termo de Consentimento Livre e Esclarecido, cabem os seguintes comentários:
   a. Ainda que tenha ficado bem claro que se trata de pesquisa de Mestrado da aluna Helga Bruxel Carvalho Follmann, orientado pela professora Eliana Elisabeth Diehl, que assina a folha de rosto como pesquisadora responsável, no TCLE está apresentado apenas o telefone institucional da pesquisadora responsável. Solicita-se que sejam apresentadas outras formas de contato com

a pesquisadora responsável, assim como número de telefone fixo da pesquisadora que irá conduzir a coleta de dados.

b. Conforme está na Resolução 304/2000: "2 – Descrição do processo de obtenção e de registro do Termo de Consentimento Livre e Esclarecido – TCLE, assegurada a adequação às peculiaridades culturais e lingüísticas dos envolvidos." Solicita-se que seja feita a adequação na linguagem dos TCLEs para cada público-alvo e versões distintas do TCLE devem ser apresentadas para cada um dos públicos-alvo a serem estudados: (a) Membros da Equipe Multidisciplinar de Saúde Indígena, (b) Técnico/Auxiliar de enfermagem; (c) Coordenadores/ Professores do curso de Técnico/auxiliar de Enfermagem e (d) Membros da Comunidade.

c. Solicitamos que o TCLE detalhe o que será requerido dos sujeitos de pesquisa, como o tempo que será necessário para a entrevista e os documentos que serão solicitados para comprovação (como citado no questionário da página 27, numeração do CEP).

5. Com relação ao orçamento:

a. Não é informado patrocinador do estudo, apenas que: "Os itens de capital, como livros, computador, impressora, gravador, entre outros, são contrapartida da UFSC ou dos pesquisadores." e que: "O projeto será submetido a Editais de fomento à pesquisa." Vale lembrar que o orçamento do projeto é peça fundamental para análise ética por significar a garantia de acompanhamento e cuidados aos sujeitos de pesquisa e por explicitar a distribuição de ônus e benefícios que devem ser objeto do julgamento ético. Além disso, deve-se evitar a descontinuação da pesquisa, segundo o item VII.13.f da Res. 196/96 "Considera-se como antiética a pesquisa descontinuada sem justificativa aceita pelo CEP que a aprovou." Ver também o item III.3."h" e "e" da Res. CNS nº 251/97. Solicita-se esclarecimento quanto ao(s) patrocinador(es) responsável(is) pela pesquisa e as garantias de que a mesma não sofrerá descontinuidade por falta de patrocínio.

Diante do exposto, a Comissão Nacional de Ética em Pesquisa – CONEP, de acordo com as atribuições definidas na Resolução CNS 196/96, manifesta-se pela aprovação do projeto de pesquisa proposto, devendo o CEP verificar o cumprimento das questões acima, antes do início do estudo.

Situação: Protocolo aprovado com recomendação.

Brasília, 29 de setembro de 2010.

Gysélie Saddi Tannous
Coordenadora da CONEP/CNS/MS

ds/lc

ANNEX 3

Authorisation from the National Indian Foundation

MINISTÉRIO DA JUSTIÇA
FUNDAÇÃO NACIONAL DO ÍNDIO

AUTORIZAÇÃO PARA INGRESSO EM TERRA INDÍGENA	N°: 90 /AAEP/10

IDENTIFICAÇÃO

ome: Helga Bruxel Carvalho Follmann	Processo: n°.1391/99
icionalidade: brasileira	Identidade: RG n°.2175777 2 SSP PR
stituição: Universidade Federal de Santa Catarina	
trocinador:	

OBJETIVO DO INGRESSO

senvolver o projeto de mestrado intitulado "A inserção do técnico/auxiliar indígena de enfermagem em uma Terra dígena Kaingang (Santa Catarina): uma análise sobre o seu papel no modelo de atenção à saúde indígena", sob a ientação da Profa. Eliana E. Diehl.

EQUIPE DE TRABALHO

Nome	Nacionalidade	Identidade
**		
**		
**		

rra Indígena: Xapecó	Etnia: Kaingang
ordenação Regional: Chapecó	Coordenação Técnica: Chapecó

VIGÊNCIA DA AUTORIZAÇÃO

cio: 09 de agosto de 2010	Término: 09 de agosto de 2011

OBSERVAÇÕES

Remeter à Assessoria de Acompanhamento aos Estudos e Pesquisas/Funai, duas cópias da monografia, relatórios, tigos, livros, gravações, imagens e outras produções oriundas do trabalho realizado.

Esta autorização não inclui cessão de uso de imagem e som de voz dos índios, nem de acesso ao conhecimento adicional associado a biodiversidade.

torizo:

Brasília, 04 de agosto de 2010.

Presidente da FUNAI
Márcio Augusto Freitas de Meira
Presidente da Funai

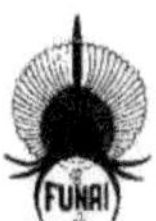

Fundação Nacional do Índio
Assessoria de Acompanhamento aos Estudos e Pesquisas
SEPS 702/902, bloco A, 3º, andar Brasília – DF CEP70390-025
telefax (61) 3313-3846 / 3313-3606 e-mail egep@funai.gov.br

Ofício nº. / 35 /AAEP/10

Brasília, 12 de agosto de 2010.

À Senhora
Profa. Eliana Diehl
Universidade Federal de Santa Catarina
Campus Universitário, B. Trindade
88040-900 Florianópolis - SC

Assunto: Ingresso em Terra Indígena (Proc. nº.139199)

1   Cumprimentando-a, estamos encaminhando original das Autorizações para Ingresso em Terra Indígena nº.90/AAEP/10 (em anexo), concedida a pesquisadora Helga Bruxel Carvalho Follmann, para ingressar na TI Xapecó, com o objetivo de desenvolver o projeto de mestrado intitulado "A inserção do técnico/auxiliar indígena de enfermagem em uma Terra Indígena Kaingang (Santa Catarina): uma análise sobre o seu papel no modelo de atenção a saúde indígena", sob sua orientação.

Atenciosamente,

Cláudio dos Santos Romero
Assessor

G MAES oficios/OF doc

ANNEX 4

Subjects - Technical Diploma in Nursing

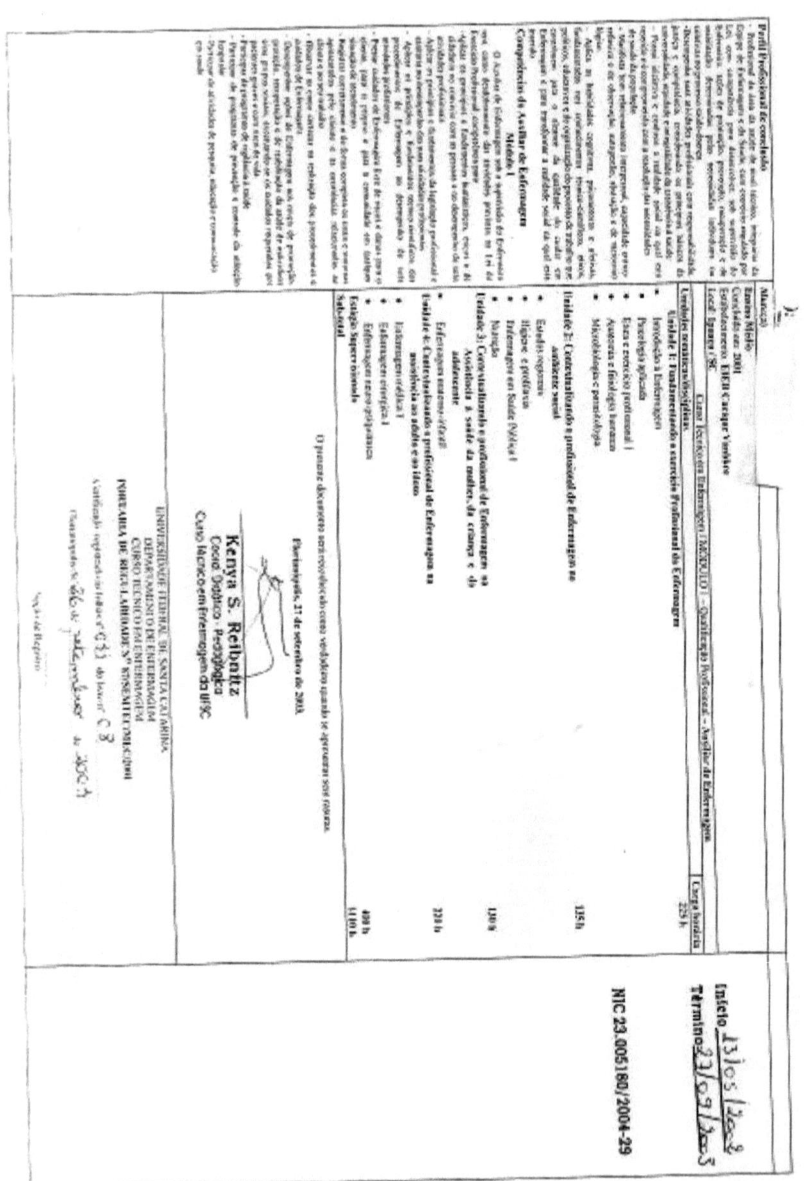

Perfil Profissional de conclusão

- Profissional da área da saúde de nível técnico, integrante da Equipe de Enfermagem e da Saúde, com exercício regulado por Lei, com competência para desenvolver, sob supervisão do Enfermeiro, ações de proteção, promoção, recuperação e de reabilitação determinadas pelas necessidades individuais ou coletivas no processo saúde-doença.
- Desempenha suas atividades profissionais com responsabilidade, justiça e competência, considerando os princípios básicos da universalidade, equidade e integralidade da assistência à saúde.
- Possui iniciativa e contribui à realidade social na qual está inserido e é comprometido com a resolução das necessidades de saúde da população.
- Manifesta bom relacionamento interpessoal, capacidade comunicativa e de observação, autogestão, educação e de motivação lógica.
- Aplica as habilidades cognitivas, psicomotoras e afetivas, fundamentadas nos conhecimentos técnico-científicos, éticos, políticos, educativos e de organização do processo de trabalho que constituem para o alcance da qualidade do cuidar em Enfermagem e para transformar a realidade social na qual está inserido.

Competências do Auxiliar de Enfermagem

Módulo I

O Auxiliar de Enfermagem sob a supervisão do Enfermeiro terá como desdobramento das atividades previstas na Lei do Exercício Profissional, competências para:

- Aplica os princípios e fundamentos humanísticos, éticos e de cidadania no convívio com as pessoas e no desempenho de suas atividades profissionais.
- Aplicar os princípios e fundamentos da legislação profissional e existente no desempenho das suas atividades profissionais.
- Aplicar os princípios e fundamentos técnicos científicos dos procedimentos de Enfermagem no desempenho de suas atividades profissionais.
- Prestar cuidados de Enfermagem livre de risco e danos para o cliente, para o próprio e para a comunidade em qualquer situação de atendimento.
- Registrar corretamente e de forma completa os dados e numeros apresentados pelo cliente e as ocorrências relacionadas ao cliente e no seu trabalho.
- Observar os como cuidados na realização dos procedimentos e cuidados de Enfermagem.
- Desempenhar ações de Enfermagem nos casos de proteção, promoção, recuperação e de reabilitação da saúde de indivíduos e/ou grupos sociais, executando-se os cuidados requeridos por pacientes graves e com risco de vida.
- Participa de programas de vigilância à saúde.
- Participar de programas de prevenção e controle da infecção hospitalar.
- Participar de atividades de pesquisa, educação e comunicação em saúde.

Marcação)	
Ensino Médio	
Concluído em: **2001**	
Estabelecimento: **EIEB Cacique Vanhkre**	
Local: **Ipuaçu /SC**	

Curso Técnico em Enfermagem / MÓDULO I – Qualificação Profissional – Auxiliar de Enfermagem	Carga horária
Unidades temáticas/disciplinas	225 h
Unidade 1: Fundamentando o exercício Profissional da Enfermagem	
• Introdução à Enfermagem	
• Psicologia aplicada	
• Ética e exercício profissional I	
• Anatomia e fisiologia humana	
• Microbiologia e parasitologia	
Unidade 2: Contextualizando o profissional de Enfermagem no ambiente social	135 h
• Estudos regionais	
• Higiene e profilaxia	
• Enfermagem em Saúde Pública I	
• Nutrição	
Unidade 3: Contextualizando o profissional de Enfermagem na Assistência à saúde da mulher, da criança e do adolescente	130 h
• Enfermagem materno-infantil	
Unidade 4: Contextualizando o profissional de Enfermagem na assistência ao adulto e ao idoso	320 h
• Enfermagem médica I	
• Enfermagem cirúrgica I	
• Enfermagem neuro-psiquiátrica	
Estágio Supervisionado	400 h
Subtotal	1110 h

O presente documento será reconhecido como verdadeiro quando se apresentar seus razoras.

Florianópolis, 27 de setembro de 2003.

Kenya S. Reibnitz
Coord. Didático - Pedagógica
Curso Técnico em Enfermagem da UFSC

UNIVERSIDADE FEDERAL DE SANTA CATARINA
DEPARTAMENTO DE ENFERMAGEM
CURSO TECNICO EM ENFERMAGEM
PORTARIA DE REGULARIDADE N° 87/SEMTEC/MEC/2001

Certificado registrado na folha n° 083 do livro C8

Florianópolis, 26 de setembro de 2004

Seção de Registro

Início 13/05/2002
Término 27/09/2003

NIC 23.005180/2004-29

Perfil Profissional de conclusão

- Profissional da área da saúde de nível técnico, integrante da Equipe de Enfermagem e da Saúde, com exercício regulado por Lei, com competência para desenvolver, sob supervisão do Enfermeiro, ações de promoção, prevenção, recuperação e de reabilitação determinadas pelas necessidades individuais ou coletivas no processo saúde-doença.
- Desempenha suas atividades profissionais com responsabilidade, justiça e competência, considerando os princípios básicos da universalidade, equidade e integralidade da assistência à saúde.
- Possui iniciativa e conhece a realidade social na qual está inserido e é comprometido com a resolução das necessidades de saúde da população.
- Manifesta bom relacionamento interpessoal, capacidade crítico-reflexiva e de observação, autogestão, abstração e de raciocínio lógico.
- Aplica as habilidades cognitivas, psicomotoras e afetivas, fundamentadas nos conhecimentos técnico-científicos, éticos, políticos, educativos e de organização do processo de trabalho que contribuem para o alcance da qualidade do cuidar em Enfermagem e para transformar a realidade social na qual está inserido.

Competências do Técnico em Enfermagem

- Aplicar os princípios e fundamentos humanísticos, éticos e de cidadania no convívio com as pessoas e no desempenho de suas atividades profissionais.
- Aplicar os princípios e fundamentos da legislação profissional e sanitária no desempenho das suas atividades profissionais.
- Aplicar os princípios e fundamentos técnico-científicos dos procedimentos de Enfermagem no desempenho de suas atividades profissionais.
- Prestar cuidados de Enfermagem livre de riscos e danos para o cliente, para si próprio e para a comunidade em qualquer situação de atendimento.
- Registrar corretamente e de forma completa os sinais e sintomas observados e relatados pelo cliente e as ocorrências relacionadas ao cliente e ao seu trabalho.
- Observar as cinco certezas na realização dos procedimentos e cuidados de Enfermagem.
- Desempenhar ações de Enfermagem, inclusive a pacientes em estado grave, nos níveis de promoção, proteção, recuperação e de reabilitação da saúde de indivíduos e/ou grupos sociais, **excetuando-se** os cuidados requeridos por pacientes internados sob risco de vida.
- Participar do planejamento, programação e orientação das atividades de assistência de Enfermagem.
- Participar da prevenção e do controle sistemático dos danos físicos decorrentes da assistência à saúde.
- Participar da prevenção e controle sistemático da infecção hospitalar.
- Atuar nos programas de higiene e segurança no trabalho.
- Participar de programas de vigilância à saúde.
- Desenvolver atividades de educação e comunicação em saúde.
- Participar de programas de pesquisa.
- Compreender o processo de trabalho da Enfermagem e da Saúde.

Disciplines - Diploma Nursing Auxiliary

Perfil Profissional de conclusão	Aluno(a):
- Profissional da área da saúde de nível técnico, integrante da Equipe de Enfermagem e da Saúde, com exercício regulado por Lei, sem competência para desenvolver, sob supervisão do Enfermeiro, ações de proteção, prevenção, recuperação e de reabilitação determinadas pelas necessidades individuais em relativas ao processo saúde-doença. - Desempenha suas atividades profissionais com responsabilidade, justiça e competência, considerando os princípios básicos da universalidade, equidade e integralidade da assistência à saúde - Possua iniciativa e conheça a realidade social na qual está inserido e é comprometido para a resolução das necessidades de saúde da população - Manifesta bom relacionamento interpessoal, capacidade crítico-reflexiva e de observação, autogestão, liderança e de responder lógico - Aplica as habilidades cognitivas, psicomotoras e afetivas, fundamentadas nos conhecimentos técnico-científicos, éticos, políticos, educativos e de organização do processo de trabalho que contribuam para o alcance da qualidade da saúde em Enfermagem e para transformar a realidade social na qual está inserido. **Competências do Auxiliar de Enfermagem** **Módulo 1** O Auxiliar de Enfermagem sob a supervisão do Enfermeiro, como desdobramento das atividades previstas na Lei do Exercício Profissional, competindo-lhe: - Aplicar os princípios e fundamentos humanísticos, éticos e de cidadania no convívio com as pessoas e no desempenho das atividades profissionais - Aplicar os princípios e fundamentos da legislação profissional e social no desempenho das suas atividades profissionais. - Aplicar os princípios e fundamentos técnico-científicos dos procedimentos de Enfermagem no desempenho de suas atividades profissionais. - Preparar unidades de Enfermagem livre de riscos e danos para o cliente, para si próprio e para a comunidade em qualquer situação de atendimento - Registrar corretamente e de forma completa os sinais e sintomas apresentados pelo cliente e as ocorrências relacionadas ao cliente e ao seu trabalho - Observar as cinco corretas na realização dos procedimentos e cuidados de Enfermagem - Desempenhar ações de Enfermagem nos níveis de prevenção, promoção, recuperação e de reabilitação da saúde dos indivíduos, dos grupos sociais, extensivos às unidades requeridas por pacientes graves e com risco de vida - Participar de programas de vigilância à saúde - Participar de programas de promoção e controle da infecção hospitalar. - Participar de atividades de pesquisa, educação e conscientização em saúde	**Ensino Médio** Concluído em: 2001 Estabelecimento: EIEB Cacique Vanhkre Local: Ipuaçu / SC

Curso Técnico em Enfermagem (MÓDULO I) – Qualificação Profissional – Auxiliar de Enfermagem	Carga horária
Unidades temáticas/disciplinas	
Unidade 1: Fundamentando o exercício Profissional da Enfermagem	225 h
• Introdução à Enfermagem	
• Psicologia aplicada	
• Ética e exercício profissional I	
• Anatomia e fisiologia humana	
• Microbiologia e parasitologia	
Unidade 2: Contextualizando o profissional de Enfermagem no ambiente social	135 h
• Estudos regionais	
• Higiene e profilaxia	
• Enfermagem em Saúde Pública I	
• Nutrição	
Unidade 3: Contextualizando o profissional de Enfermagem na Assistência à saúde da mulher, da criança e da adolescente	130 h
• Enfermagem materno-infantil	
Unidade 4: Contextualizando o profissional de Enfermagem na assistência ao adulto e ao idoso	330 h
• Enfermagem médica I	
• Enfermagem cirúrgica I	
• Enfermagem neuro-psiquiátrica	
Estágio Supervisionado	490 h
Sub-total	1110 h

O presente documento será reconhecido como verdadeiro quando se apresentar com carimbo.

Florianópolis, 27 de setembro de 2003.

Kenya S. Reibnitz
Coord. Didático - Pedagógica
Curso Técnico em enfermagem da UFSC

UNIVERSIDADE FEDERAL DE SANTA CATARINA
DEPARTAMENTO DE ENFERMAGEM
CURSO TÉCNICO EM ENFERMAGEM
PORTARIA DE REGULARIDADE Nº 87/SEMTEC/MEC/2001

Certificado registrado às folhas nº (3) sob nº 03

Reconhecido ... de setembro de 2003

Seção de Registro

ANNEX 6

UFSC graduation photos

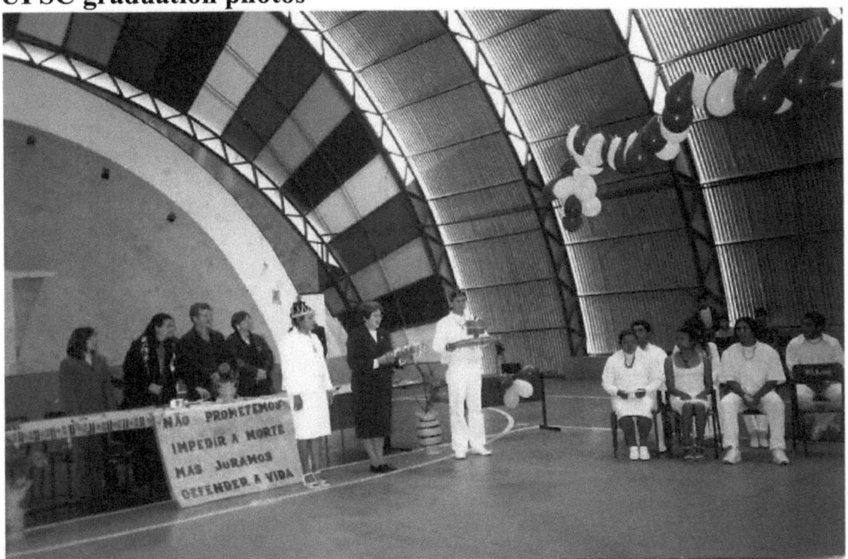

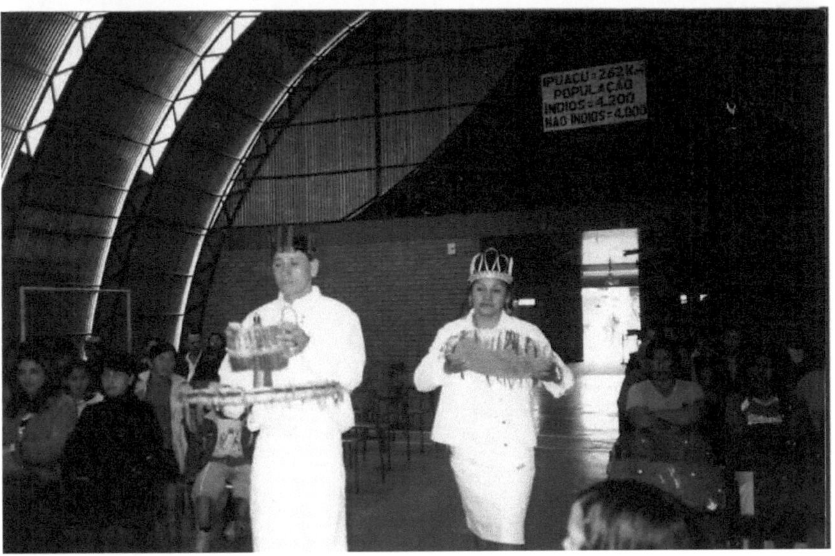

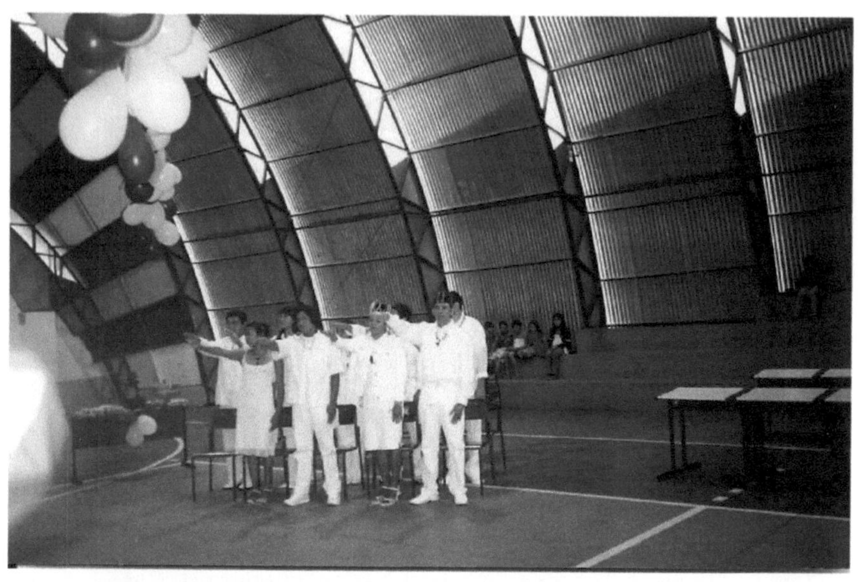

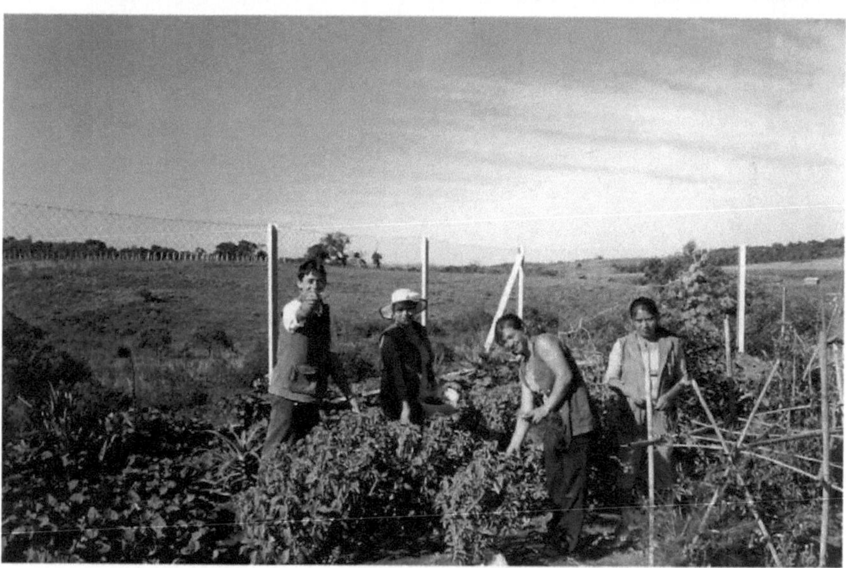

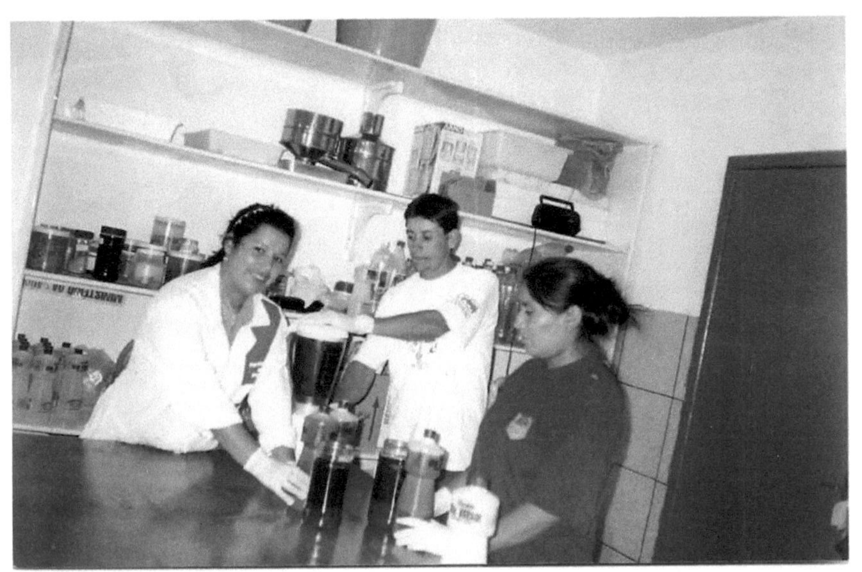

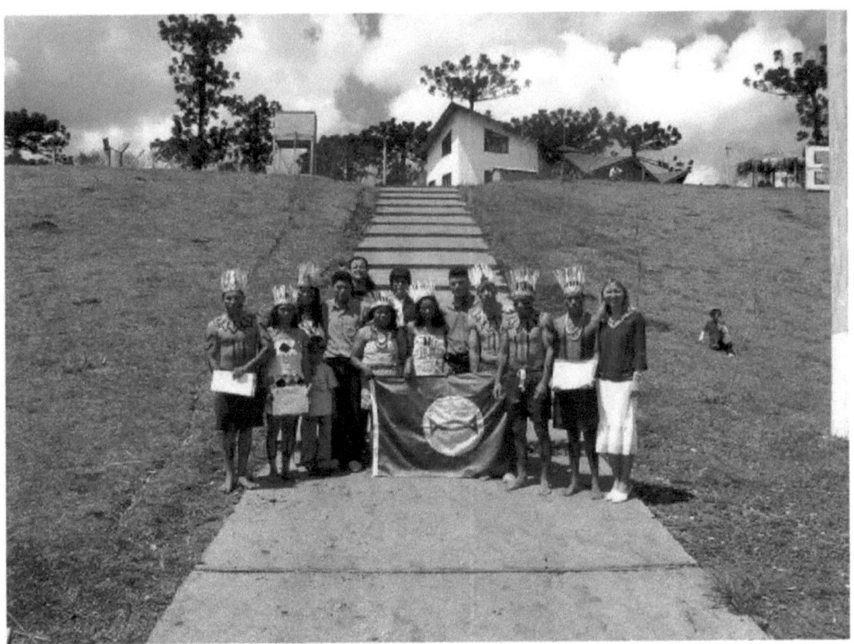

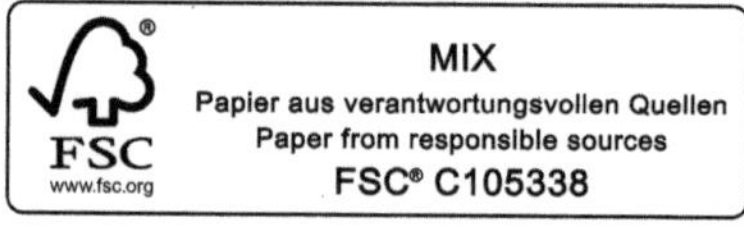

Printed by Books on Demand GmbH, Norderstedt / Germany